Smart Guide™
to
Getting Thin and Healthy

About Smart Guides™

Welcome to Smart Guides. Each Smart Guide is created as a written conversation with a learned friend; a skilled and knowledgeable author guides you through the basics of the subject, selecting out the most important points and skipping over anything that's not essential. Along the way, you'll also find smart inside tips and strategies that distinguish this from other books on the topic.

Within each chapter you'll find a number of recurring features to help you find your way through the information and put it to work for you. Here are the user-friendly elements you'll encounter and what they mean:

The Keys

Each chapter opens by highlighting in overview style the most important concepts in the pages that follow.

Smart Money

Here's where you will learn opinions and recommendations from experts and professionals in the field.

Street Smarts

This feature presents smart ways in which people have dealt with related issues and shares their secrets for success.

Smart Sources

Each of these sidebars points the way to more and authoritative information on the topic, from organizations, corporations, publications, web sites, and more.

Smart Definition

Terminology and key concepts essential to your mastering the subject matter are clearly explained in this feature.

F.Y.I.

Related facts, statistics, and quick points of interest are noted here.

What Matters, What Doesn't

Part of learning something new involves distinguishing the most relevant information from conventional wisdom or myth. This feature helps focus your attention on what really matters.

The Bottom Line

The conclusion to each chapter, here is where the lessons learned in each section are summarized so you can revisit the most essential information of the text.

One of the main objectives of the *Smart Guide to Getting Thin and Healthy* is not only to better inform you about how to start a weight-loss program, but to make you smarter about nutrition and foods to ensure a lifetime of healthful benefits.

Smart Guide™

to

Getting Thin and Healthy

Katharine Colton

CADER BOOKS

John Wiley & Sons, Inc.

New York • Chichester • Weinheim • Brisbane • Singapore • Toronto

Library of Congress Cataloging-in-Publication Data:
Colton, Kitty.
Smart guide to getting thin and healthy / Kitty Colton.
p.   cm.   — (Smart guide)
Includes bibliographical references and index.
ISBN 0-471-29634-1
1. Weight loss. 2. Nutrition. 3. Health. I. Title. II. Series.
RM222.2.C573   1998
613.2'5—dc21   98-33832

Printed in the United States of America

10 9 8 7 6 5 4 3 2 1

Contents

Introduction .... *ix*

1. No-Bull Guidelines for Successful Weight Loss **1**
1. Decide to Change Your Lifestyle 2
   Dieting versus Healthy Eating 3
   What about Willpower? 4
   The Health Factor 4
2. Educate Yourself 5
   The Role of Genetics 7
3. Go for the Goal—but Be Realistic 8
   To Weigh or Not to Weigh? 8
   An Alternative to Scale Watching 9
4. Listen to Your Body 9
   When to Eat? 10
   Alert Eating 10
5. Think Moderation, Not Denial 11
6. Take It Slow 13
   How Fast Should You Lose? 14
   The Thyroid Connection 14
7. Be Adventurous 14
   Shopping Safari 15
8. Don't Go It Alone 15
9. Exercise, Exercise, Exercise 16
   Changing Your Set Point 17
   No Sweat? 18
   Pleasure Counts More Than Calories 19
   Weights and Weight Loss 20
Every Step You Take 21
   Variety Is Key 22

2. Where to Start **23**
Are You Ready to Lose? 24
   Why You Should Think Twice about Dieting 25
   The Wrong Time to Lose 25
   The Right Reason for Change 26
Evaluating Your Weight 27
   Why the Scale Can Be Misleading 29
   The Body Mass Index 29
   Why Your Body Shape Matters 32
   The Body Fat Factor 32
   How to Measure Your Fat 33

How Many Calories Should You Consume? 35
   What to Cut 37
Keeping a Food Diary 37
   What to Record 41
Should You Do It Yourself? 42
   Pros and Cons of Weight-Loss Centers 43

3. Fats, Proteins, and Carbohydrates **45**
Why It Pays to Bone Up 46
The Three Basics: Fats, Proteins, and Carbohydrates .. 48
Fat Facts 48
   The Down Side 49
   Bad and Good Fats 49
      The Bad 50
      The Good 50
   How Much Fat Should You Eat? 51
   Why Less Fat Isn't Always Better 52
   The Perils of Cholesterol 53
   The Good and Bad News about Reduced-Fat Foods .. 54
Protein Facts 56
   How Much Do You Need? 57
   Complete versus Incomplete
   Proteins, and Where to Find Them 57
      The Vegetarian Way:
      Combining Proteins 58
   What about High-Protein Diets? 59
Carbohydrate Facts 59
   Simple versus Complex 60
   Good and Not-So-Good Sugars 62

4. Noncaloric Nutrients **63**
Vitamins and Minerals 64
   Vital Vitamins 64
      Vitamins 65
   Do You Need a Supplement? 68
   Vital Minerals 69
      Minerals 70
      Spotlight on Calcium 72
Good and Bad Sodium 74
Two Other Essentials: Fiber and Water 75
   Fiber Facts 76
   Water Wisdom 77
      How Much Do You Need? 78

5. The Best Foods **79**
The Food Guide Pyramid 80
   Serving Sizes 82
   How Many Servings Should You Eat? 83
The Pyramid's Smart Foods 87
   Bread, Cereal, Rice, and Pasta 88
      Best Bets: Bread Group 88
   Fruit and Vegetable Groups 90
      Best Bets: Fruit 92
      Best Bets: Vegetables 94
   Dairy Group 97
      Best Bets: Diary Group 97
   Protein Group 101
      Best Bets: Animal Proteins 101
      Best Bets: Vegetable Proteins 103
   Fats, Oils, and Sugars 107
      How Much Fat? 107
      Cutting the Fat 108
      Making Trade-Offs 109
      A Word about Chocolate 109

6. Eating Smart Every Day **111**
Supermarket Savvy 112
   Essential Reading 113
   Deciphering Labels 114
      Serving Size, Servings per Container,
      Calories per Serving 114
      Calories from Fat per Serving 114
      % Daily Value 115
      Protein and Other Nutrients 116
   Nutritional Claims 117
   Fresh Food Tips 117
The Joy of Cooking Thin 122
   Some Simple Rules 122
   Cutting the Fat 124
Putting It All Together 126
Healthy Menus to Get You Started 128
   Breakfast Menus 128
   Lunch Menus 129
   Dinner Menus 130
   Healthy Snacks and Add-Ons 131
   Small Meals 132
The Pyramid Plan 134
   Checklist for Healthy Menus 136
   Daily Eating Do's and Don'ts 136

7. Danger Zones **139**
The Pleasures and Perils of Eating Out 140
   Restaurant Roulette 141
   Dining-Out Strategies 142
   More Tips for Smart Dining 143
      The Bread Basket 143
      Appetizers and Salads 144
      Entrées 145
      Vegetables 145
      Dessert 146
      Beverages 147
   Fast Food 147
   Eating on the Run 148
   Snacking and Good-Time Eating 149
Fun Food 150
Snacking in Solitude 153
   Trigger Foods 154
When Healthy
Eating's Not a Family Affair 155
   What to Watch For 156
The Lowdown on Drinking 156
Mood and Food 157

8. Weight Loss That Lasts **159**
Hitting a Plateau 160
   Adjusting Your Expectations 162
   Knowing When to Stop 162
Keeping It Off 163
   Mapping Out a Maintenance Plan 164
   Working without a Net 165
Staying Motivated 166
   Giving Yourself a Break 167
Bouncing Back from a Lapse 167
Reality Check 168
A Final Note 169

Appendix: Calories and Fat for Selected Foods *170*
   Breads, Cereals, and Grains *170*
   Fruits *171*
   Vegetables *172*
   Dairy *173*
   Meat, Poultry, Eggs, Seafood, and Legumes *174*
   Fats, Oils, and Salad Dressings; Nuts and Seeds *176*
Index *177*

Introduction

Some people trying to lose extra weight look for "miracle" diets, but you are smart enough to know that they don't exist. The *Smart Guide to Getting Thin and Healthy* doesn't spin myths or insult your intelligence. Here, you won't find a radical new eating plan of seaweed and pomegranate seeds. What you will find is a whole lot of commonsense advice in a no-jargon, no-gimmick form.

Simply put, weight loss and healthy weight maintenance consists of two ingredients: mind and matter.

It works like this: First, you decide to adopt a smart, healthy lifestyle. Now and forever. That's the mind part. Then you put that thought into action by choosing the foods, and adopting the day-by-day changes and habits that will fit your new mindset and get you to your goals. That's the matter.

Putting it simply doesn't mean it's a simple task. Losing weight and keeping it off is in no way easy; if it were, those truckloads of diet books wouldn't keep flying off the shelves—one of them long ago would have revealed the secret to painless dieting. But the fact is getting and staying slim is like everything else worth doing: It takes effort. The good news is that what starts out as a tough proposition indeed—changing what may be a lifetime of bad habits—gets easier and easier as you go along. Two things work in your favor, neither of which is magic but both of which come close: the huge psychological lift you'll get from losing weight and adopting a healthy lifestyle; and the new, healthier habits and cravings your body will adopt over time.

Although there are no shortcuts to weight loss and better health, you can cut through the diet hokum and hype and get to the facts. The *Smart Guide to Getting Thin and Healthy* tells you what you need to know to reach and maintain a healthy, happy weight. Period.

In chapter 1 you'll learn the basic tenets of successful weight loss—guidelines that won't just get you thin but that will also keep you that way for a lifetime. Chapter 2 helps you examine your old eating habits and set the stage for new ones.

To become a savvy eater, you need to know what's in what you're eating. Chapters 3 and 4 give you the lowdown on fat, protein, carbohydrates, vitamins, and all other nutritional basics. Once you get smart to nutrition, you'll be able to make your own wise choices instead of blindly following some boring weight-loss regimen.

In chapters 5 and 6 you'll find out which foods give you the most nutritious bang for your caloric buck. Then you'll learn how to shop and cook wisely—and get a head start on your own menu planning with some sample meal plans.

Chapter 7 guides you through the diet danger zones: parties, restaurant meals, and other potential hazards. A few strategic eating tips will help you relax and enjoy rather than binge and regret. Finally, chapter 8 helps ensure that all your hard work won't go to waste: You'll learn how to maintain your new weight and your new healthy habits and how to bounce back from dietary setbacks.

As with human relationships, so it is with food relationships: Even smart people can make foolish choices. This book aims to show you a better way. It's not about a diet; it's about a new way of eating, and a new way of life, that you can live with—happily, healthily, and, yes, thinly—forever.

No-Bull Guidelines for Weight Loss

THE KEYS

• A new mind-set, not just a new menu, is what matters most for a lifetime at an appropriate weight.

• Your body needs a variety of foods to keep in top form. Learn what it needs, and wants, to eat.

• A slow, moderate approach to weight loss is the key to long-term success.

• Finding support and seeking adventure are just two ways to help keep you on track.

• Exercise is vital to weight loss and well-being; you simply cannot afford to sit there.

You've surely seen enough how-to-do-anything-in-a-just-a-few-easy-steps lists to know they're a bit too pat and simplistic to be true. The guidelines in this chapter are not intended to condense everything there is to know about weight loss and healthy eating advice into a few bite-size chunks; nor are they black-and-white rules about what you absolutely must or mustn't do. Instead, they are intended as *guides* to help you achieve your weight-loss and weight-maintenance goals.

This chapter encompasses the big picture; you'll find answers to nuts-and-bolts, how-do-I . . . weight-loss questions in later chapters. Following these guidelines will give you a solid, sensible, smart foundation for overhauling your attitude toward food—which *is* the definitive first step toward successful weight loss. Deciding to take that step—and subsequent steps toward becoming healthier and slimmer—is up to you.

1. Decide to Change Your Lifestyle

The difference between weight-loss efforts that work and those that don't is not measured in M&Ms. Yet even some of the smartest people will swear it all comes down to that—whether we are able or unable to "deny" ourselves what's "bad" and stay on the path of virtue.

The real difference between success and failure, not only in dieting but in almost any endeavor you can name, is attitude. Successful weight loss requires a whole change in consciousness. Of course, in the short term, changing your consciousness is no easier than denying yourself a piece of cheesecake. But in the long term, it means you'll be able to eat without suffering, without denial, without fear, because you'll naturally gravitate to the foods that are good for you and make you feel your best.

Rethinking your attitudes and your behaviors, and then changing them, isn't something you do during a coffee break. It takes time, just as it took you time to build up a repertoire of unhealthy habits. It's natural to be impatient for results when you decide to lose weight and get in shape, but that cliché about the virtues of patience never held truer than now.

Dieting versus Healthy Eating

The "diet" mentality doesn't work. When the word *diet* is used in this book, it refers to all the foods you eat, not a specific, prescribed regimen. A healthy way of life is not about denial. When you start thinking of food not as your enemy—or shelter from life's storms—but as your friend, your whole outlook changes. Instead of "depriving" yourself of the foods you love, think in terms of positive choices—deciding to eat nutritious, healthy foods because you want to, because they make you feel (and look) your best.

SMART MONEY

"Turn on the mental switch that says you are going to lose weight," says Donn Jasura of the Diet and Weight Loss Home Page. "You have to *want* to lose weight. If you don't want to lose weight, forget it. You can't do it for someone else. If you really care about your health and longevity, your looks and your family, then you should have no problem turning on the switch."

You can reach the Diet and Weight Loss Home Page at: http://www.mhv.net/~donn/diet.html.

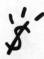

What about Willpower?

When their latest diet fails, most people place all the blame on—themselves. "I just don't have the willpower" is the common refrain. This is good news for diet-book authors, who offer up ridiculously stringent, impossible-to-maintain weight-loss plans but are not held responsible when those plans don't yield the promised miracles. But this is very bad news for dieters. When you undertake the challenge of changing your eating habits, the last thing you need is a negative, self-blaming attitude. And chalking up every slipup to lack of willpower is draining, self-defeating, and simply wrong.

A sensible, long-term eating plan is not dependent on willpower but rather on motivation. What's the difference? Willpower implies that you are, through sheer strength of character, going to stop yourself from eating the "wrong" foods. Motivation means you choose not to eat nonnutritious foods on a regular basis because they don't make you feel your best, period. And if you do reach for a few empty calories now and then, you don't beat yourself up for it. Because it doesn't represent a colossal collapse of willpower, you don't spiral into despair and start eating everything in sight; you go out for a walk and come home and have a salad and feel fine. You're motivated to stay on track.

The Health Factor

One of the best ways to get yourself thinking in terms of lifestyle changes, not quick-fix diets, is by focusing on your health, not the numbers on the bathroom scale, not even on how you look in your jeans. As you learn and become more aware of all the life-extending and quality-of-life benefits that a nutritious, balanced, low-fat diet brings, it begins to get a lot easier to pass on those artery-clogging, nonnutritious foods.

2. Educate Yourself

That's what this book is for. In the following chapters you'll learn the basics of nutrition and why certain foods are more healthful than others—which ones fuel your body and which ones do nothing for you at all. There's no need to memorize the Food Guide Pyramid (discussed in chapter 5) or a specific list of "good" and "bad" foods, but a basic brushup on nutrition is an excellent foundation; soon you'll be making healthy choices intuitively.

The more you learn about how your body works, and why it responds the way it does when you feed it too much or too little, or the wrong proportions of various nutrients, the less likely you are to grow frustrated by the "mysteries" of your body—such as why the fat on your thighs refuses to budge—and give up on your weight-loss resolve altogether. And the less likely you are to fall prey to fad diets and gimmicks that at best will result in only short-term weight loss—and at worst will seriously imperil your health.

Losing weight gradually on a balanced diet may not sound as exciting as "Drop ten pounds in five days!" or the myriad other claims you'll find in fad diet books or on the labels of weight-loss products. But here's the simple truth: Gimmicks

STREET SMARTS

"I think the most important part of the weight-loss process is learning to love yourself, regardless of your flabby thighs, before you set any diet and fitness goals," says thirty-two-year-old graduate student Drew Ewing. "When you stick to those goals, you'll be doing it because it will help the body you love, instead of working against the body you hate."

Mini-Motivators

Thinking about changing your diet and lifestyle is one thing; doing it is another. When you need a motivational jump start to keep your good intentions on track, try one of the following:

• Carry a picture of yourself, pre–weight loss, in your wallet. Or, even better, if you are really into self-confrontation, on your refrigerator.

• Make a list of reasons you want to lose weight. This might include anything from "I want to fit into the bikini I bought ten years ago" to "I want to get in shape for the next marathon." Put it next to a picture of yourself on your fridge.

• Pick up a copy of the latest health publication and read any one of the fifty articles on the dangers of being overweight.

and shortcuts don't work. That includes fasting, liquid diets, diet pills, and any eating plan that advocates strictly limiting your food choices or calorie intake. The only way to achieve long-lasting weight loss, and avoid the dreaded yo-yo dieting syndrome, is by adopting a sensible eating plan that you can live with for life.

There are several reasons that fad diets and weight-loss gimmicks are bound to backfire:

1. You can stand to eat cabbage soup (or cucumbers and rice, or whatever the latest fad dictates) for only so long. Then you are bound to rebel—not just against cabbage but against dieting altogether.

2. Depriving your body of sufficient calories slows down your metabolic rate. When you are not consuming enough food, your body goes into "starvation mode," trying to conserve whatever energy stores it has left. When this happens, it becomes nearly impossible to lose weight, no matter how little you are eating. In addition, your deprive your body of the essential nutrients it needs to keep you healthy.

3. Subsisting on juice for a week, or taking appetite suppressants, or eating bizarre food combinations does not teach you how to eat in the real world. In fact, any of these methods will leave you only more out of touch with your appetite and your ability to discern when you are hungry and what your body needs—both crucial to lasting weight loss and health.

Maybe you are one of the many people who blame their diet failures on lack of "willpower." You're doomed to repeat the same patterns unless you arm yourself with the facts about nutrition and smart, sensible eating. If you want to make a lifelong change, don't look for shortcuts.

The Role of Genetics

You've probably heard of the so-called fat gene. The term refers to the role that heredity plays in your body size and shape. It's true that you may have a genetic predisposition toward being overweight. According to Michael Myers, a doctor specializing in weight control and the treatment of obesity and eating disorders, there's approximately a 75 percent chance that the biological children of an overweight mother will also be overweight. It works the other way as well: If the mother is thin, there's a 75 percent chance that her children will be, too.

But that doesn't mean you inherit fatness. Although it is easier to gain weight if you have this genetic predisposition, you are not "destined" to be heavy. Only eating more calories than you burn will make you heavy. So don't let the fat gene get you down, and don't use it as an excuse to stay heavy. Instead, let it inspire you to beat the odds. Fat does not have to be your fate.

STREET SMARTS

"I think the problem is that people try to lose weight for a special occasion. When the occasion is over, it's back to the bad habits. You have to make a change in the way you eat and exercise for the rest of your life if you want to be fit and look great for the rest of your life," advises forty-three-year-old theater manager Don Lowe.

SMART DEFINITION

Metabolic Rate
The amount of energy (calories) the body uses each day, determined by three factors:

1. Basal metabolic rate (BMR), the minimum amount of energy required to keep the heart, brain, and other organs functioning while you are at rest

2. Energy burned during physical activity

3. Energy burned during digestion

3. Go for the Goal— but Be Realistic

You're not going on another old-fashioned, deprivation-centered diet, but that doesn't mean you shouldn't set some goals. Goals help you get where you want to go and see the results of your efforts. Plus reaching them gives you a reason to celebrate, which will provide further reinforcement.

So if you want to, go ahead and choose a goal weight. In chapter 2 you'll learn how to choose a weight that's sensible for you, not someone else. Your target weight should take into account your body type. You shouldn't aim for the low end of your healthy weight range if you have a big-boned frame. And remember, aiming for supermodel slenderness isn't what healthy eating is about. Your ideal weight should be one you can live with for life, not one that requires a deprivation diet.

Set yourself short-term goals along the way to your target weight. When you meet them, reward yourself with a nonfood treat.

To Weigh or Not to Weigh?

It's perfectly okay to weigh yourself while you're trying to lose weight. In fact, seeing the numbers go down can be a great incentive to stick to your goals. But you shouldn't take it too far. Stepping on the scale every day can do more to discourage than encourage you; water retention, for example, may signify something to your scale, but it shouldn't signify anything to you. If you want to measure your progress by the numbers, do it no more than once a week. The best way to measure your progress, however, is by how you feel and what you see in the mirror.

If you know you always get discouraged when you see those numbers glaring up at you, yet you can't keep from looking, throw the scale out.

An Alternative to Scale Watching

While it's important to get your weight within a healthy range (see chapter 2), you should not feel compelled to pick a particular target weight unless you want to. Some people feel motivated by such a tangible goal, and very satisfied when they reach it. But if you are someone who has struggled with gaining and losing (and gaining again) in the past, it may be time to forget this type of goal. Focus instead on learning to eat normally and feeling content with yourself. It's much more important than some magic number on a scale. And you're likely to find that when you stop obsessing about every pound, it's much easier to reach and maintain a healthy weight.

4. Listen to Your Body

Learn to eat only when you are hungry. Your brain triggers appetite. Yet most people eat for so many reasons other than hunger, chief among them habit and mood. Eating out of habit rather than hunger almost guarantees that you will eat more calories than you need.

SMART SOURCES

These two titles offer useful information about breaking the yo-yo dieting cycle:

Outsmarting the Female Fat Cell
Debra Waterhouse

Intuitive Eating: A Recovery Book for the Chronic Dieter
Evelyn Tribole and Elyse Resch

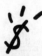

SMART MONEY

"A reasonable weight is one that you can maintain without undue suffering, at which you feel quite good about the way you look, and at which you have no serious medical problems caused by weight," informs Anne M. Fletcher, registered dietitian and author of *Thin for Life: 10 Keys to Success from People Who Have Lost Weight and Kept It Off.*

A college student who succumbed to the famous "freshman fifteen" chalks up her weight gain not to stress but to regimented eating. "Living on campus, we are scheduled to eat at certain times between classes, whether or not we're hungry," she says. "Later on, when we really *are* hungry, we gorge on candy bars and other snacks." Plenty of office workers could provide similar testimonials.

When to Eat?

Depending on your body type, activity level, and metabolism, you may want to eat the traditional three meals a day, or four to six smaller meals. Grazing—eating small portions every couple of hours—can help you keep your energy up and stave off hunger pangs (and the binges that often follow). See what works best for you. (And see chapters 6 and 7 for more on the benefits and dangers of snacks and small meals.) Do beware, though, that while small meals may be smart, it's harder to keep tally of how much you're eating that way.

Alert Eating

Paying attention to what you eat is fundamental to successful weight loss and the best way to pay attention to your food intake is by making eating a separate activity. Don't get distracted by eating in front of the TV or while reading. When you eat and only eat, you can recognize the signals your stomach is sending to tell you when you've had enough. If a sitcom laugh track drowns those signals out, you're bound to overeat.

Pay attention, too, to the way you feel when you eat nutritious foods as opposed to empty calories. It's not a matter of "virtuous" versus "guilty." It's a matter of feeling healthy and energized rather than slow and sleepy. And it's also about knowing *why* you're eating what you're eating. Are you bored? Tired? Anxious? More often than not we grab snacks for reasons other than hunger. (For more on the relationship between mood and food, see chapter 7.)

Above all, eat slowly. It's healthier. And it gives your stomach time to tell your brain you're full.

5. Think Moderation, Not Denial

Eating smart does not mean restricting yourself to broccoli and lentils, to high-fiber and low-fat, to sugar-free and salt-free and fun-free. Eating smart means choosing foods that will make you feel your best, give you energy, keep you at a healthy weight. Often it means opting for a healthier substitute to replace your old standbys—a variation on having your cake and eating it, too. Again, the more you know about nutrition, and the more you listen to your own body when it cries out for sweets, or salt, or crunch, the better you'll know how to respond with foods that are satisfying and smart at the same time.

Smart eating is easier than you think. For example, maybe it's Sunday morning, and you wake up wanting something slightly indulgent.

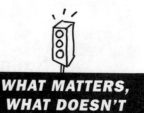

WHAT MATTERS, WHAT DOESN'T

What Matters

- Adopting a whole new mind-set.

- Learning what's healthy.

- Taking a long-term approach.

What Doesn't

- Fixating on the details.

- Swearing off everything that's not healthy.

- Judging and evaluating your every move.

Smart Substitutions That Add Up

Here are just a few examples of no-pain food switches that can save you calories—and often fat and excess sugar, too.

Instead of . . .	Try . . .
16 ounces of sweetened iced tea 220 calories	16 ounces brewed iced tea with 2 teaspoons of sugar 32 calories
1 cup premium ice cream 600 calories	1 cup premium sorbet 240 calories
12 ounces of cola 152 calories	12 ounces flavored seltzer water 0 calories
1 cup cream of chicken soup 190 calories	1 cup chicken noodle soup 75 calories

Because you're now thinking before you eat, you don't automatically reach for that package of French toast in the freezer; instead you opt for the whole-grain waffles, which you know offer fewer calories and more nutrients. Soon this sort of decision will not involve lengthy deliberations; it will become second nature. Best of all, it really doesn't involve sacrifice—just substitution of one (smarter, healthier, but otherwise similar) food for another (not so smart, not so healthy) food.

But eating smart doesn't always mean substituting. Once in a while you should allow yourself to eat whatever you *want*, period, be it an ice cream cone, a hot dog, or a slice of pepperoni pizza. Just make sure it's something that will really satisfy you, and enjoy every bite. That's the way to avoid a sense of deprivation and keep your cravings in control.

6. Take It Slow

It's worth remembering that patience is an essential ingredient in any lifestyle change—particularly one aimed at weight loss. What happens when you try to lose weight fast by eating too little? You may be all too familiar with the syndrome. You shed pounds quickly, only to gain them back just as quickly. And then you find it twice as hard to lose those same pounds the next time. If so, you're hardly alone.

Here's the scientific explanation for this distressing phenomenon: When you embark on an extremely low-calorie diet, your body goes into negative nitrogen balance, a condition that causes your body to break down muscle tissue for fuel. When you lose even a pound of muscle this way, it can mean a drop of up to 50 calories in your metabolic rate; in other words, your body may burn 50 fewer calories a day. In a nutshell, extreme diets send your body into starvation mode, slowing down its metabolism to conserve body fuel and use fewer calories. What that means is that although you may be eating next to nothing, you will be losing nothing, either. And the metabolic damage will last into your next diet, and the one after that, and on and on.

How Fast Should You Lose?

One-half pound to a pound a week, or 1 percent of your body weight, is a manageable, healthy rate. If you grow impatient with the slow-but-steady approach, remember this: When you shed pounds gradually, you're more apt to lose fat than muscle or water.

The Thyroid Connection

Another problem with very-low-calorie diets is that they interfere with a chemical produced by your thyroid to regulate body temperature. If your thyroid isn't producing enough of this chemical, your metabolic rate will slow down, and you'll suffer the weighty consequences.

If you have used an extreme diet to lose weight, you'll have to wean yourself back to regular eating to avoid rebound weight gain. Depending on how severe the diet was and how long you were on it, it can take up to three months of carefully monitoring your diet and gradually increasing calories so you can resume normal eating habits and return your thyroid levels to normal.

7. Be Adventurous

Your attitude toward food should be the same as your attitude toward life: To get the most out of both, you have to be willing to try new things. Your local supermarket probably offers a vast array of foods you've never heard of, let alone eaten. It's likely there are others you tried once, perhaps as a child, and instantly hated—and you've never touched them since. (Vegetables such as brussels sprouts often fall in this category.) When you make a decision to get out of your food rut, you'll find a world of undiscovered or over-looked choices to replace the tired old standbys.

Shopping Safari

Make shopping an event. Make a point of adding one new fruit, vegetable, grain, or legume to your cart each time you go shopping; buy something you know nothing about, then look for a fun new recipe in which to use it. You'll find there are hundreds more uses for fresh produce and whole grains than for processed convenience foods.

Even if you're adamantly anti-cooking, there's plenty of ready-to-eat exotica out there. Kiwifruit, for example. Any new fruit or vegetable is bound to be a bonus to your diet. (See chapter 5 for a list of top bangs—exotic and everyday—for your nutritional and caloric buck.)

The key is to think opportunity, not oppres-sion. For every food you're better off without, there's a new healthy one waiting to be discovered.

8. Don't Go It Alone

Of course, losing weight and getting healthy is ultimately up to no one but you.

But support can make a world of difference. That doesn't mean you need to join a formal group such as Weight Watchers, with its member-

Have You Tried . . . ?

Adzuki beans

Bok choy

Collard greens

Couscous

Fresh figs

Guavas

Millet

Papayas

Parsnips

Swiss chard

ship fees and scheduled meetings. (For more on the benefits and pitfalls of such programs, see chapter 2.) Friends or family can do the trick as well. If you can establish a buddy system with a friend or a spouse, you'll both get a boost from the mutual support. People who have succeeded in losing weight will be delighted to share their tips, too—witness Oprah Winfrey.

Sometimes the support will be there waiting for you, arms wide open. Close friends and loved ones who have supported you in the past may be just the ones to help you now. Or they may not. Many people benefit from networking with others who are trying to lose weight, too. If you're lucky, you may know a friend or coworker who fills the bill. If not, try your health club—ask around or post a notice. Whether you just want to share recipes or find a workout partner, you are most definitely not alone.

9. Exercise, Exercise, Exercise

If you want to lose weight, you've got to expend more calories than you consume. Yes, you can do this without exercising, but not efficiently, smartly, or healthfully. Exercising makes losing weight infinitely easier, not just because you're burning more calories on the court than on the couch, but also because working out gives you a physical and a mental—even a spiritual—boost that improves your outlook and attitude, and thus your chances of achieving success at whatever you do—including the matter at hand, eating right and getting in shape.

This is another realm in which mind and matter must work together. If you make a conscious decision to incorporate more activity into your life because you want to feel and look better, you will have the positive motivation to make it happen.

The key, as with a healthy diet, is to start out small and incorporate new activities gradually. Don't push yourself too much, too soon, if you're more accustomed to hiking to the fridge than up a mountain.

Changing Your Set Point

According to the "set point" theory, your body works to keep your weight at a certain level. No matter how much weight you gain or lose, your body will adjust the number of calories it burns in order to bring your weight back to its set point.

If you've lost weight and then regained it despite your best intentions, this theory may sound wholly credible to you. And there's research to back it up: The *New England Journal of Medicine* reports on a study that shows adults who gained weight after overeating burned more calories, which suggests that their bodies were trying to return to their usual weights. Underfed adults who lost weight used fewer calories.

Sounds pretty hopeless, eh? But wait—here's the good news: If a set point does exist, exercise may be the key to changing it. Say you want to lose fifteen pounds. You start cutting calories and the weight comes off. According to the set point theory, your body will then lower its energy use. But if you start to exercise regularly, the calories you burn will offset the set point adjustment, so you stay at your new lower weight.

STREET SMARTS

Going it alone can be rough when you're trying to lose weight and exercise. Twenty-seven-year-old kindergarten teacher Denise Newburg has this advice to ensure success: "Get a weight-loss, fitness buddy—someone to weigh in with, exercise with, compare notes with. The competition and camaraderie definitely help!"

"Try to establish a set time each day to exercise," advises forty-six-year-old advertising executive Lucinda Simon. "I make exercise a part of my daily routine, just like brushing my teeth. I've grown to think of it as a way of life, not as a chore. Anything you think of as a chore will eventually fall by the wayside."

No Sweat?

One of the most heartening pieces of health news to emerge in recent years is that mild to moderate exercise is just as good for you as the vigorous, sweaty kind. In some ways it's even better. This is the kind of exercise that's impervious to such excuses as "I don't have time to go to the gym" or "My knees give out when I run." Ideally you will have time in your life for sustained activity, be it swimming or biking, tennis or the treadmill—but if you don't, you can still incorporate more movement into your daily routine. And it all adds up. Contrary to what we were once told, it doesn't matter whether you walk for thirty minutes every morning or for ten minutes three times a day. It's the total amount of exercise that counts, not the duration of each workout.

However, if you want to lose a significant amount of weight, the best way to do so is with regular, sustained aerobic exercise (the kind that gets your heart pumping), combined with weight training (more on that later). The American College of Sports Medicine in Indianapolis recommends cardiovascular exercise three to five days a week at 60 to 90 percent of maximum heart rate for twenty to sixty continuous minutes, expending at least three hundred calories per session.

If you do decide to take up a vigorous activity, go slow at first. Especially if you've started cutting calories, your body may have a hard time adjusting, and you'll end up tired and discouraged instead of energized. And always see a doctor before you begin a new exercise program.

Pleasure Counts More Than Calories

It's natural to want to know how many calories you're burning, but you shouldn't obsess about it.

Wise Workouts

Here's the calorie-burning lowdown on some favorite activities and calories burned per 20 minutes.

Activity	120 lbs.	140 lbs.	160 lbs.	180 lbs.
High-impact aerobics	148	172	196	220
Basketball	150	176	200	226
Biking (10 mph)	110	128	146	164
Golf (carrying clubs)	92	108	124	140
Hiking	90	104	120	134
In-line skating	118	138	158	176
Jogging	186	216	248	278
Running	228	264	302	340
Skiing (cross-country)	150	176	200	226
Skiing (downhill)	114	132	152	170
Swimming (moderate pace)	156	180	206	232
Tennis	120	138	158	178
Walking	120	152	174	194
Weight training	132	152	174	196

F.Y.I.

Walking a mile and a half each day at a fairly brisk pace (in thirty minutes) will result in a weight loss of two pounds in a month without any reduction in calories.

Find the kinds of exercise that you enjoy and that make you feel good—the ones that rev you up, energize you, relieve stress. These are the activities you'll want to stick with. Again, just as with eating, we are talking long-term here. Exercise should not be used as a shortcut to weight loss; it should become part of the fabric of your life, as natural a part of your day as your morning shower.

Weights and Weight Loss

Even those who are sold on the weight-loss and maintenance benefits of exercise often overlook a crucial component: strength training. That's a big mistake. Working out with weights is as crucial as aerobic exercise to your health; just two twenty-minute sessions a week will maintain your muscles and bones and help prevent back pain. The bonus: Strength training is also a great calorie-burning and metabolism-raising tool. Plus whatever weight you're carrying is going to look better on you when you improve your muscle tone.

The American College of Sports Medicine recommends the following as a minimum twice-weekly strength-training regimen: one set (eight to twelve repetitions) of eight to ten exercises that condition the major muscle groups. If you join a gym, you'll get instructions on how to use the weight-training equipment, such as Nautilus or Cybex. Don't try to figure it out for yourself! You're likely to waste valuable time straining the wrong muscles altogether; even small mistakes in positioning and form can mean the difference between a great workout and a pointless one. It's also easy to hurt yourself on this stuff, whether by straining a ligament or dropping a weight on your toe.

Every Step You Take

There may be times when you're too busy for a full-fledged workout. But don't make that an excuse—you can still incorporate some physical activity into even the most hectic day. One frazzled but fit executive advises, "Maximize the exercise and calorie-burning potential of every little thing you do. Instead of taking the elevator, take the stairs. If you talk on the phone a lot, get a cordless phone and pace around the house while you chat." Here are some other painless ideas:

• When you drive to a store, park at the far end of the lot.

• If you take the bus or subway to work, get off a stop or two before your destination and walk briskly the rest of the way.

• Do isometrics at your desk or at the movies (double benefit: It is very hard to do isometrics and eat popcorn simultaneously). When you exhale, pull your stomach in quickly and tightly and push the air out. Slowly let your stomach out as you breathe in.

• Break up a daily walk into small, manageable chunks—ten minutes before work, ten at lunch, ten after work in the evening.

SMART SOURCES

For guidelines on exercise and fitness:

Aerobics and Fitness
  Association of
America
15250 Ventura Blvd.
Suite 200
Sherman Oaks, CA
  91403-3297
800-225-2322
http://www.afaa.com

American Council on
  Exercise
5820 Oberlin Drive
Suite 102
San Diego, CA 92121-
  3787
619-535-8227
http://www.
acefitness.org

Variety Is Key

Cross-training is based on the idea that you can't get a complete workout by doing any one exercise over and over. Different kinds of exercise tackle different body parts: Walking, for instance, is great for your legs; swimming builds endurance and conditions your arms as well. Varying your routine whips more of you into shape, faster, and it helps prevent injuries to boot.

And it makes exercise more fun—which is crucial. Alternating workouts keeps you engaged and challenged, which means you're likely to keep at it. Just as with your diet, the same old same old can be the kiss of death when it comes to keeping on the exercise track. Think of new activities as spices added to the fitness mix.

If you're aiming to lose weight, try alternating a couple of favorite cardiovascular activities for your recommended minimum weekly workout (three to five times a week, for twenty to sixty minutes), adding a couple of strength-training sessions each week.

THE BOTTOM LINE

Long-term weight loss and weight maintenance requires an overhaul not just of your refrigerator but of your outlook and lifestyle. Before you can succeed, grasp the basics: A realistic attitude, nutritional know-how, and a motivated mind and body are the foundations for success.

CHAPTER 2

....

Where to Start

You can probably figure out whether you need to lose weight simply by looking in the mirror or trying on last year's (or last decade's) jeans. But it's not so simple to figure out how much you need to lose—or how to start doing it.

This chapter includes charts and numbers that give you information on how much you should weigh, how much excess fat you're carrying around, and what daily calorie level will help you get rid of it. Such facts and figures will help you assess your health and fitness level and target a safe, efficient weight-loss strategy. But before you start assessing your physique, take a minute to examine your psyche.

Are You Ready to Lose?

Losing weight isn't just a numbers game. You may already know how much you want to lose, and have a good idea of what it will take to do so, but that doesn't mean you're ready to start. No amount of information will be useful to you if you aren't mentally ready to undertake a new way of eating and living. Here are some factors you should consider before launching a new weight-loss effort.

Why You Should Think Twice about Dieting

Not only is repeat dieting damaging to your morale, but it's also hard on your figure—and your health. Losing and regaining weight again and again—the yo-yo dieting syndrome—damages your metabolism and makes each subsequent weight-loss effort more difficult. Furthermore, the well-known Framingham Heart Study, cited in the *New England Journal of Medicine* in 1991, reported that people who diet frequently suffer from coronary heart disease more often than nondieters and died sooner, usually from heart problems.

This information is not intended to discourage you from embarking on a weight-loss effort but to make you consider whether you are ready to begin. And we're not talking about beginning another short-term, quick-acting diet that's doomed to end in failure, we're talking about a whole new healthy lifestyle.

The Wrong Time to Lose

You should always check with your doctor before starting on a weight-loss plan. And if you are pregnant, don't even think about it. There are other times when you shouldn't consider losing weight, either:

• When you are making another big change in your life (such as moving, changing jobs, starting graduate school) that requires all your energy;

SMART MONEY

Anne M. Fletcher, author of *Thin for Life: 10 Keys to Success from People Who Have Lost Weight and Kept It Off*, offers this sound advice: "The possible negative consequences of yo-yo dieting suggest *not* that you should give up your effort to lose weight, but that you should take a long, hard look at how serious you are before you make your next attempt at weight loss."

• When you are dealing with a stressful situation (such as caring for a new baby, going through a divorce);

• When you are feeling sad or depressed.

You might be tempted to add losing weight to your agenda during many of these times. Perhaps you figure that since you're already starting one new project, it's a great time to start another. Or you think concentrating on losing weight will lessen your stress. Or you attribute your blues to your excess weight.

Those are all reasonable theories, but the reality is that most weight-loss efforts undertaken in times of duress or depression are bound to fall by the wayside. Changing your eating and exercise habits is hard enough under optimal conditions; don't make it harder by undertaking it while you're distracted or stressed out. Above all, don't try to change your lifestyle while you're feeling down; while it's true that your weight problems may be adding to your dark mood, you should wait till you're in a more positive frame of mind to start dealing with them. Be patient; when the time is right, you'll know it.

The Right Reason for Change

One more caveat: Never start a new eating and exercise plan unless you can say the following with complete honesty: *I am doing this for myself.*

That means you are not trying to lose weight in order to catch someone else's attention or approval or to fit anyone else's standards.

It may sound like a cliché, but it's absolutely true: You have to want to change for yourself.

True motivation, the kind that makes you achieve your goals, comes from within. And remember, where eating and good health are concerned, you are setting lifetime goals, not the kind that last only through your class reunion or your ex-boyfriend's upcoming party.

If you're confident you're ready to begin, then read on!

Evaluating Your Weight

Most people over- or underestimate how much they need to lose. That's where weight charts and other measuring devices come in.

Health professionals sometimes use the following simple formula to determine average weights:

• **For women:** Begin with a height of 5 feet and a weight of 100 pounds. Add 5 pounds for every inch of height over 5 feet. Then calculate 10 percent of this total; adding or subtracting that figure gives you your healthy weight range. If you have a small frame, subtract 10 percent; if you have a large frame, add 10 percent. For example, if you are five foot four, your healthy weight averages 120 pounds, with a range of about 12 pounds up or down.

• **For men:** Begin with a height of 5 feet and a weight of 106 pounds. Add 6 pounds for every inch of height over 5 feet. Use the method above to determine your weight range.

You can also simply check a weight chart such as the one below, which lists healthy weight ranges for adults.

Healthy Weight Ranges for Men and Women

Height	Weight (in pounds)	Height	Weight (in pounds)
4'10"	91–119	5'9"	129–169
4'11"	94–124	5'10"	132–174
5'0"	97–128	5'11"	136–179
5'1"	101–132	6'0"	140–184
5'2"	104–137	6'1"	144–189
5'3"	107–141	6'2"	148–195
5'4"	111–146	6'3"	152–200
5'5"	114–150	6'4"	156–205
5'6"	118–155	6'5"	160–211
5'7"	121–160	6'6"	164–216
5'8"	125–164		

Source: Dietary Guidelines for Americans, 1995 ed., U.S. Department of Agriculture, U.S. Department of Health and Human Services

Why the range? Because people of the same height may have equal amounts of body fat but different amounts of muscle and bone. Keep in mind that these weights are guidelines; they aren't set in stone. If you check various weight charts you will find a variety of ranges, though they generally vary by only a few pounds.

Why the Scale Can Be Misleading

Although the importance of keeping your weight within a healthy range—or getting it back there—can't be overemphasized, there are limits to what your scale can tell you. As noted above, the ranges given for each height are meant to accommodate a variety of body types, including those more or less muscular. Your muscle mass makes a difference because muscle weighs more than fat.

If you begin a new workout routine, particularly one that involves weight training, you may be dismayed to find your weight increasing rather than decreasing. But don't get discouraged! This merely means you are converting some of your body fat to muscle. Even though it may not look good on the scale, it will look great on your body. That's why you should judge your success by how your clothes fit and how you look in the mirror instead of relying exclusively on the scale.

The Body Mass Index

To determine if you are overweight, you need to assess more than just your weight. Your body mass index (BMI) is a measurement of your weight in relation to your height, based on a mathematical formula that correlates with your body fat. Specifically, it's determined by calculating your weight in kilograms divided by your height in meters squared. This number is a better predictor of disease risk than body weight alone.

To determine your BMI, check the following chart, and note:

SMART MONEY

"I don't aspire to look like Kate Moss; I don't aspire to being as smart as Einstein, either, but that's no excuse for not being my best," says Susan Estrich, legal scholar and author of *Making the Case for Yourself: A Diet Book for Smart Women.*

• A BMI of 24 or less means you are at minimal health risk. An acceptable BMI means your weight is not putting you at increased risk for health problems such as heart disease, diabetes, and some types of cancer.

• The World Health Organization and other major health organizations classify "overweight" as a BMI of 25 or over.

Body Mass Index

Weight	115	120	125	130	135	140	145	150	155	160	165
Height											
5'0"	22	23	24	25	26	27	28	29	30	31	32
5'1"	22	23	24	25	26	26	27	28	29	30	31
5'2"	21	22	23	24	25	26	27	27	28	29	30
5'3"	20	21	22	23	24	25	26	27	27	28	29
5'4"	20	21	22	23	24	25	26	27	27	28	29
5'5"	19	20	21	22	22	23	24	25	26	27	27
5'6"	19	19	20	21	22	23	23	24	25	26	27
5'7"	18	19	20	20	21	22	23	23	24	25	26
5'8"	17	18	19	20	21	21	22	23	24	24	25
5'9"	17	18	18	19	20	21	21	22	23	24	24
5'10"	17	17	18	19	19	20	21	22	22	23	24
5'11"	16	17	17	18	19	20	20	21	22	22	23
6'0"	16	16	17	18	18	19	20	20	21	22	22
6'1"	15	16	16	17	18	18	19	20	20	21	22
6'2"	15	15	16	17	17	18	19	19	20	21	21
6'3"	14	15	16	16	17	17	18	19	19	20	21
6'4"	14	15	15	16	16	17	18	18	19	19	20

• A BMI of 30 or more means you are at a serious health risk.

• Bodybuilders and professional athletes, pregnant or lactating women, and sedentary elderly people are not good candidates for BMI measurements due to atypical bone mass, muscle mass, and fluid levels.

Weight	170	175	180	185	190	195	200	205	210	215	220
Height											
5'0"	33	34	35	36	37	38	39	40	41	42	43
5'1"	32	33	34	35	36	37	38	39	40	41	42
5'2"	31	32	33	34	35	36	37	37	38	39	40
5'3"	30	31	32	33	34	35	35	36	37	38	39
5'4"	29	30	31	32	33	33	34	35	36	37	38
5'5"	28	29	30	31	32	32	33	34	35	36	37
5'6"	27	28	29	30	31	32	32	33	34	35	36
5'7"	27	27	28	29	30	31	31	32	33	34	34
5'8"	26	27	27	28	29	30	30	31	32	33	33
5'9"	25	26	27	27	28	29	30	30	31	32	32
5'10"	24	25	26	27	27	28	29	29	30	31	32
5'11"	24	24	25	26	26	27	28	29	29	30	31
6'0"	23	24	24	25	26	26	27	28	28	29	30
6'1"	22	23	24	24	25	26	26	27	28	28	29
6'2"	22	22	23	24	24	25	26	26	27	28	28
6'3"	21	22	22	23	24	24	25	26	26	27	27
6'4"	21	21	22	23	23	24	24	25	26	26	27

Source: World Health Organization

Why Your Body Shape Matters

Where extra weight settles on your body makes a difference. Research has shown that if you are an "apple" shape, carrying extra fat in your stomach area, you're at greater risk for high blood pressure, diabetes, early heart disease, and some kinds of cancer than if you're a "pear" shape, carrying more fat in your hips and thighs. If you can't tell by a glance in the mirror, you can use a measuring tape to determine your waist-to-hip ratio:

1. Measure your waist where it's narrowest; don't suck in your stomach while doing so.

2. Measure your hips at their widest point.

3. Divide your waist measurement by your hip measurement to get your waist-to-hip ratio.

The ideal for women is 0.8 or below; for men, it's 0.95 or less. Don't panic if you discover you're an apple: The good news is, it's often easier to lose fat around the abdomen than around the hips and thighs. Aerobic exercise and a low-fat diet are the prime weapons.

The Body Fat Factor

Another, more accurate way to assess your health and fitness level is by measuring your body composition—the ratio of fat tissue to lean. Your ideal weight is your lean body mass (everything but fat) plus just enough fat for good health—18 to 25 percent of total body weight for women and 10 to 18 percent of total body weight for men. No matter what you weigh, if your body fat is beyond that range, you are overfat.

How to Measure Your Fat

There's no absolutely precise way to measure your body fat, but there are three techniques that come pretty close:

• **Hydrostatic weighing,** the most accurate method, involves underwater weighing; it's based on the principle that muscle is denser than fat and therefore weighs more underwater. However, it's usually done only at research facilities because of equipment and space requirements.

• The **percent body fat test,** the most commonly used method, measures skin-fold fat thickness with a caliper. This method is based on the fact that about 50 percent of body fat is found just under the skin; health professionals measure skin folds on various parts of the body and put those measurements into an equation to determine total body fat. Many fitness clubs offer these tests when you join.

• **Bioelectrical impedance** involves passing a small electrical current through the body, using electrodes placed on the skin. Because fat impedes electrical currents more than muscle does, the "impedance value" can be used to estimate the percent of body fat.

Both the percent body fat test and bioelectrical impedance are good ways of measuring changes in your body composition over time, but they may not detect small changes in fat. If your BMI and waist-to-hip ratio are healthy, there's probably no need to worry. Otherwise, you should work at replacing fat with muscle, both by exercising (weight training is especially effective) and by following the kind of healthy, balanced eating plan outlined in the following chapters. Remember: Most restrictive diets cause you to lose both lean and fat body weight; a slow-but-steady approach will help you maintain your lean tissue while reducing the fat.

Calories Needed Daily

Women

Height	Healthy Weight	Sedentary	Moderately Active	Active	Extremely Active
4'11"	95	1,045	1,235	1,425	1,710
5'0"	100	1,100	1,300	1,500	1,800
5'1"	105	1,155	1,365	1,575	1,890
5'2"	110	1,210	1,430	1,650	1,980
5'3"	115	1,265	1,495	1,725	2,070
5'4"	120	1,320	1,560	1,800	2,160
5'5"	125	1,375	1,625	1,875	2,250
5'6"	130	1,430	1,690	1,950	2,340
5'7"	135	1,485	1,755	2,025	2,430
5'8"	140	1,540	1,820	2,100	2,520
5'9"	145	1,595	1,885	2,175	2,610
5'10"	150	1,650	1,950	2,250	2,700
5'11"	155	1,705	2,015	2,325	2,790
6'0"	160	1,760	2,080	2,400	2,880

How Many Calories Should You Consume?

It doesn't get more basic than this: The way to lose extra body fat is by eating fewer calories than you take in each day. The best way to do this is not by counting every calorie you put in your mouth, but rather by eating the foods that are good for you and naturally low in calories and fat—and by exercising.

Men

Height	Healthy Weight	Sedentary	Moderately Active	Active	Extremely Active
5'2"	118	1,298	1,534	1,770	2,124
5'3"	124	1,364	1,612	1,860	2,232
5'4"	130	1,430	1,690	1,950	2,340
5'5"	136	1,496	1,768	2,040	2,448
5'6"	142	1,562	1,846	2,130	2,556
5'7"	148	1,628	1,924	2,220	2,664
5'8"	154	1,694	2,002	2,310	2,772
5'9"	160	1,760	2,080	2,400	2,880
5'10"	166	1,826	2,158	2,490	2,988
5'11"	172	1,892	2,236	2,580	3,096
6'0"	178	1,958	2,314	2,670	3,204
6'1"	184	2,024	2,392	2,760	3,312
6'2"	190	2,090	2,470	2,850	3,420
6'3"	196	2,156	2,548	2,940	3,528
6'4"	202	2,222	2,626	3,030	3,636

Source: The HOPE Heart Institute, Seattle, Washington

Calories and Metabolism

Your daily calorie needs vary based on two factors:

• Your basal metabolic rate (BMR)—the number of calories your body needs while at rest

• Your normal activity level

A chart can give you an estimate of how many calories you need per day, depending on your activity level, but it's likely you'll need to adjust the figure up or down to fit your own metabolism. You can estimate your BMR by multiplying your current weight (in pounds) by 10 if you're a woman or 11 if you're a man. For example, if you're a woman who weighs 120 pounds, you require about 1,200 calories a day just to keep your body functioning. You also need some percentage of calories above your BMR to provide energy for your daily activities. That figure varies widely, depending on your metabolism and activity level. If you're moderately active, you might need 30 to 50 percent more calories to maintain your weight; at 120 pounds, that would mean approximately 1,680 calories per day (1,200 + [1,200 × .40] =1,680). If you're trying to lose weight, aim for the number of calories needed to maintain your ideal (not current) weight. Most health-care professionals recommend that women take in at least 1,200 calories per day (1,400 for adolescent girls, 1,600 for men); if you go below that, you won't get sufficient nutrients and you will risk sending your body into "starvation" mode.

To estimate how many calories your body needs to maintain its current weight, both at rest and in action, multiply your BMR by the activity level that best fits you:

1.3 Sedentary (normal everyday activities; no vigorous exercise)

1.4 Moderately active (exercise three to four times a week)

1.6 Active (exercise more than four times a week)

1.8 Extremely active (exercise an hour or more six to seven times a week)

The more active you are, the more calories you'll burn; for example, if you replace your sedentary lifestyle with an active one, you'll burn almost 25 percent more calories (that's 500 or so!).

However, even if you don't plan to count calories religiously (and you're better off if you don't), it's useful to have a target calorie range when you're starting a weight-loss program. Once you get under way and develop a good sense of what to eat and in what amounts, you can ignore these numbers; you'll soon be attuned to what your body needs without having to check figures and charts.

Though it's impossible to measure precisely how many calories you are burning each day, you can start with a reasonable estimate and then adjust your intake and activity level if you aren't losing weight. The chart on pages 34–35 can help you determine how many calories you need to reach or maintain your ideal weight. (The weights are averages; if you have a small or large frame, adjust these figures up or down.)

What to Cut

To lose weight at a healthy pace, cutting fat rather than lean tissue, you should start by reducing your daily caloric intake by about 300 calories. You'll learn about healthy ways to do that in the coming chapters. If you also increase your physical activity to burn off about 200 extra calories a day, you can easily burn more than 3,500 calories a week—a pound's worth. That's the rate most nutritionists consider healthy.

Keeping a Food Diary

Recording every bite you eat and every sit-up you do may sound like a colossal waste of time, and doubly

SMART SOURCES

The mother of all nutrition organizations is a fertile source of healthy information:

American Dietetic
    Association
216 West Jackson
    Blvd.
Chicago, IL 60606-
    6995
312-899-0040
http://www.eatright.org

so if lack of time's a big reason you eat poorly and barely get to the gym in the first place. But keeping a food and activity diary is well worth a few minutes of time and effort each day. Here's why:

• Keeping a record forces you to think about what you eat. Even if you think you know how many calories you consume each day, you are more than likely forgetting myriad little bits and bites you unwittingly put in your mouth between meals, on the run, at the movies, and on and on it goes. If you continue on this path, your weight-loss efforts are doomed to end in frustration.

What's Your Eating Pattern?

You may be surprised (pleasantly or not at all) by what a food diary reveals about your habits. In a study published in the *American Journal of Clinical Nutrition*, David Schlundt, a psychology professor at Vanderbilt University who specializes in nutrition issues, asked a group of women who were entering weight-loss programs to keep a food diary for two weeks before the programs began and again during the programs. Along with their food intake, they were asked to record their perceptions and behaviors at each meal, including whether they craved sweets, were tempted to overeat, whether forbidden foods were available, and who prepared the meal.

Although all the women in Schlundt's study reported that their diets contained excess fat, the researcher detected five distinct patterns of eating behavior among them:

• **Restrained eaters.** Those who control their eating habits carefully but have a low metabolic rate and find they can't lose weight. Many such people are victims of the yo-yo diet syndrome. The prescription: Gradually increase calorie and exercise levels to raise metabolism; stop obsessing about every bite.

• **Moderate eaters.** Those who eat fairly normally and make healthy choices but tend to overeat at meals. The prescription: Increase physical activity to lose weight; learn to substitute low-fat foods for high-fat ones.

• Writing everything down helps you make a connection between what you eat and why you eat it. You may well be completely oblivious to the connection between what you eat, when you eat it, and how you feel at the time, but there's often a direct link between mood and food, and seeing it in black and white can help you detect patterns and break the habit of eating for reasons other than hunger.

• A record enables you to see how active you really are—and it's quite likely you're less active than you think.

STREET SMARTS

"People tell me not to lose weight—I might lose my personality. I tell them, 'Honey, my personality ain't in my thighs.'"
—Oprah Winfrey

• **Alternating diet/binge eaters.** Those who, like restrained eaters, are obsessed with limiting food intake but respond to emotional stress by bingeing. The prescription: Stop dieting and learn to eat according to natural appetites; learn new ways of coping with emotions.

• **Emotional overeaters.** Those who, unlike diet/binge eaters, *regularly* eat too much in stressful situations. They aren't obsessed with controlling their food intake, but they do have trouble controlling their emotions. The prescription: Focus on learning to dealing with emotions and on separating food and mood.

• **Unrestricted meal overeaters.** Those who consistently eat a high-fat, high-calorie diet. People in this group, says Schlundt, eat whatever they want whenever they want it, without any apparent connection to emotions. The prescription: Learn to eat a low-fat, lower-calorie diet; therapy might help provide motivation.

You may find that you fall into more than one of these groups, or into a different group at different times of your life. What the classifications really prove, says Schlundt, is that people relate to food in a variety of ways. Keeping a diary can help you determine your own particular patterns and weaknesses; only by recognizing them can you begin to change them.

Eating and Exercise Diary

	Time	What I ate	Where I ate	My mood	Hunger level (1–5)
Breakfast					
Lunch					
Dinner					
Snacks					
	Time	What I did	How long	My mood	Hunger level (1–5)
Exercise					

Perhaps you're continually puzzled when you find you've put on another few pounds despite your "good" eating and exercise habits. Keeping a diary for a week or two—weekends included!—will help you identify the specific dietary culprits that are keeping you from losing pounds or making you pile on more of them. Basically, it's a very efficient way of making you confront your real habits and start changing them.

It may not be pleasant to record those two candy bars you inadvertently nibbled after dinner, but doing so makes you accountable for your behavior—and makes you think twice before doing the same thing again.

If you're going to go to the trouble of trying to change your habits, you don't want to waste your time by committing acts of self-sabotage and then conveniently "forgetting" them. You need to learn that what you eat counts, even if you eat it in front of the refrigerator; and whether you actually went to the gym one or four times this week counts, too. It all adds up.

So start writing it all down. Examining your behaviors and patterns is the first step toward establishing new, healthier ones.

What to Record

Your diary should include information on where, when, and how much you ate or drank, and how you were feeling at the time. (Hungry? Depressed? Bored?)

If you are already physically active or starting up a new exercise program, devote a section of your diary to this as well. Look for correlations between your activity levels and eating habits.

STREET SMARTS

"I didn't have much to lose, but I was a closet eater. If someone didn't see me eat it, it didn't have calories." Cathy Calhoun, a fifty-two-year-old nurse has this advice: "Writing down everything I ate made every bite real. I clearly saw how much I was consuming. There were still days when I overate—including bingeing on a big bag of cookies—but I wrote it all in my diary anyway, and the next day I went right back to healthy eating."

SMART SOURCES

Here's where to lodge complaints or find information about weight-loss products and programs:

Consumer Response Center
Federal Trade Commission
6th St. and Pennsylvania Ave., NW
Washington, DC 20580
202-326-3128
http://www.ftc.gov

These could be either encouraging or discouraging. Do you tend to eat more as a reward for working out? Or do you find that your workouts put you in such a good mood that you have no trouble with overeating?

After a week or so of this, you may be able to write down what you eat before you eat it, which in itself may curb your appetite considerably.

Should You Do It Yourself?

The stage is set:

• You've determined that you're ready to lose weight.

• You've figured out your target weight range and calorie level.

• You've set the starting date and have marked it on your calendar.

• You've started keeping a diary to monitor your eating and exercise habits.

The next step is to learn a new, healthier way of eating. It's not complicated or demanding; as a matter of fact, you can learn everything you need to know in the pages of this book. But it does require some self-discipline and motivation.

That's one reason many people turn to weight-loss groups such as Weight Watchers when they decide to change their eating habits—they want structure and support. For many people, such groups can provide just that; others find they can achieve longer-lasting change on their own.

Whichever plan works best for you, remember that your determination and positive approach throughout the process will be a few keys to your success.

Pros and Cons of Weight-Loss Centers

According to the Food and Drug Administration, approximately 8 million Americans a year enroll in some kind of structured weight-loss program. All of the established weight-loss organizations— Weight Watchers, Jenny Craig, Nutri-System, and the like—offer reliable information, balanced nutritional plans, and counseling, plus the comfort of belonging to a group. If the idea of going it alone sounds daunting, and you know you do better in a structured environment, you might want to consider joining a center. But before you do, consider the following:

• The Federal Trade Commission has challenged the overblown claims of several weight-loss companies. It's a good idea to check with the FTC before signing up with any program—and putting your money and your health on the line.

• Ask the weight-loss organization for data that proves its program works—over the long haul. (Published studies indicate that relatively few participants in weight-loss programs manage to keep the weight off long-term.)

• Ask about any health risks; check with your doctor to make sure the plan is healthy and safe, and if there are any health risks involved.

• Find out the costs for membership, fees, food, supplements, maintenance, and counseling, and when these need to be paid. Make sure you know whether you can get a refund if you're dissatisfied.

• Ask about the counselors' credentials.

One warning: If you are tempted to try a weight-loss program to provide a quick-fix solution and save you the trouble of implementing real, lasting changes in your lifestyle, please think twice. No matter how supportive it may be, a program cannot always be there to motivate you and tell you what to do. The fundamental will to lose weight and get healthy has to come from within. If you decide to join such a group, think of it as a tool, not a crutch.

THE BOTTOM LINE

Weights and measures and calorie counts have their place, but nothing is as important to a successful weight-loss plan as feeling ready, physically and mentally, to commit yourself to a new, healthier way of life. After assessing your current health level and deciding on a reasonable weight-loss goal, you need to take an honest look at what's been keeping you from that goal in the past so you can learn to change those patterns.

CHAPTER 3

Fats, Proteins, and Carbohydrates

THE KEYS

• Understanding nutrition basics will make a difference not only in your weight-loss efforts but in your health.

• Not *all* fat is bad, but not knowing the good fats from the bad fats (and which to enjoy and which to avoid) could hinder your progress.

• All bodies need protein, and how much is determined by your own unique factors; like most things in life, too much of it is not a good thing.

• Hands down, the foundation of a healthy diet and the best fuel source for your body are the carbohydrates.

• Sugar can be found in many different forms. By whatever name, sugar is best in moderation.

You may think nutrition is something to worry about later, after you've lost weight. After all, it's hard enough just dealing with calorie counts—never mind all that stuff about food groups and fiber and minerals and vitamins. Anyway, you feel pretty confident about the basics: Fat is bad, protein is good, and carbohydrates are—good? Bad? Maybe you're not quite sure, come to think of it. Which is understandable, considering the mixed messages that bombard you daily via the latest diet books, news reports, your office mates . . .

Well, you can always pop a pill or two to provide all the nutrition you need. Right?

Wrong.

Granted, when you set out to lose weight, it's very easy to forget about everything but how much you're consuming. But it's not smart. Nor is operating on vague assumptions about what you should and shouldn't be feeding your body.

Why It Pays to Bone Up

Ignoring nutrition in your quest for thinness can be a fatal mistake (sometimes literally). The smart thing to do is to learn the ABCs of good nutrition, because looking and feeling your best isn't just about restricting calories; it's about knowing what to put in your body in order to get the best out of your body. And the more you learn about the nutrients and other essential elements that fuel and fortify you, the more you'll be able to make the right choices for a lifetime of thin, healthy eating. When you grasp the basics of good nutrition, those choices will soon become second nature, not dependent on the artificial strictures of one fad diet or another.

Speaking of which, a solid foundation in the roles of fat, protein, and carbohydrates can go a long way toward clarifying which diet plans are legitimate, which are sheer hocus-pocus, and which, if you follow them, could endanger your life. Arming yourself with nutritional knowledge puts *you* in control, and that's the key to weight loss and weight maintenance, now and forever.

Don't worry: You don't need to return to school for a degree in nutritional chemistry. Most of this stuff is pretty elementary; what matters is learning to be aware of what your body needs and why, which will help you when you're:

• Trying to decipher food labels at the market;

• Choosing vitamins at the health-food store;

• Deciding whether you're better off eating cantaloupe or kumquats.

Best of all, learning about nutrition may help open your eyes—and palate—to a whole new world of food possibilities. Nature conveniently arranged for many of the most nutritious foods to be wonderful weight-loss and weight-maintenance allies as well.

SMART SOURCES

These two books offer an abundance of information about nutrition and healthy eating:

The Nutrition Bible
Barbara Deskins and
    Jean E. Anderson

*The American Dietetic
    Association's
    Complete Food and
    Nutrition Guide*
Roberta Larson Duyff

SMART DEFINITION

Calorie
A unit of energy contained in food. Four components in food provide calories:

• Fat—provides 9 calories per gram.

• Protein—provides 4 calories per gram.

• Carbohydrate—provides 4 calories per gram.

• Alcohol—provides 7 calories per gram.

The Three Basics: Fats, Proteins, and Carbohydrates

Everyone's familiar with these nutrients. And you probably have your own set of (maybe vague) ideas about which are good and which are bad. Every year, it seems, various weight-loss gurus spring up like weeds to tell you that protein is king or carbs are key. But there's one perennial refrain: Fat makes you fat.

That's a good place to start setting the nutritional record straight.

Fat Facts

So *does* fat make you fat? Well, yes and no. Fat is the most concentrated form of energy you can consume. It provides more than twice as many calories per gram as protein or carbohydrates—which is the number-one reason dieters, in particular, are eager to shun it. And it's true that by limiting fat intake alone, you are likely to reduce, at least somewhat, your total calorie intake.

But although you wouldn't know it from listening to the myriad nonfat zealots out there, fat is *essential* to your body. Eliminating all fat from your diet is just about impossible—and a very bad idea to boot. You don't need much fat in your diet, but you must consume some. In addition to giving you energy, fat supplies essential fatty acids and enables your body to process and store the fat-soluble vitamins A, D, E, and K. Furthermore, fat helps keep your hair and skin from drying out, helps you sleep at night, and helps regulate mood. So despite what diet gurus like Dean Ornish may say, fat is not The Enemy.

The Down Side

The big problem with fat—the reason fat makes you fat—is that it tastes so good you end up eating way more than you need. And your body quickly takes any excess fat and stores it, quite securely, as body fat. That can lead not only to obesity but a number of other serious health threats as well, including arterial clogging and heart disease—even cancer. No wonder that in survey after survey, consumers consistently rate fat their top nutrition concern. But no matter how much weight you want to lose, you shouldn't try to cut out fat entirely—just carefully monitor your intake, and particularly watch what *kind* of fat you're taking in.

Bad and Good Fats

Many fat-phobes don't realize that there are good and bad kinds of fat. The difference comes down to fatty acids, the basic chemical units in fat. Fatty acids are molecules made up mostly of carbon and hydrogen. The more hydrogen they contain, the more saturated they are. Saturated fats contain the most hydrogen; polyunsaturated fats contain the least.

F.Y.I.

The top energy-producing nutrient is fat, not carbohydrates.

**WHAT MATTERS,
WHAT DOESN'T**

What Matters

• Eating good unsaturated fats.

• Reducing intake of saturated fats and trans fats.

• Keeping overall fat consumption to 30 percent of your diet or less.

What Doesn't

• Obsessing about high-cholesterol foods (unless you have very-high-cholesterol levels).

• Eating fat-free or reduced-fat foods that are still loaded with empty calories.

• Trying to eat a very-low-fat diet in order to lose weight.

The Bad

Saturated fat. It's found in meat, high-fat dairy foods, tropical oils (such as coconut oil and palm kernel oil), and hydrogenated (solidified) vegetable oils. Saturated fat is the kind you should strive to minimize because:

• It's linked to cardiovascular disease;

• It causes blood cholesterol to rise.

Lately scientists have pinpointed another kind of bad fat, called "trans" fat, which makes up 5 to 10 percent of the fat in American diets. Trans fat is a "hybrid" fat made by adding hydrogen atoms to a polyunsaturated fat to make it more saturated. Found in most margarine, commercial baked goods, and foods deep-fried using hardened vegetable oils, trans fat is listed on food labels as hydrogenated or partially hydrogenated fat.

The Good

Unsaturated fat. Unsaturated fats include **monounsaturated fat**, which is missing one pair of hydrogen atoms, and **polyunsaturated fat**, which lacks more than one pair of hydrogen atoms. Monounsaturated fats include olive oil, peanut oil, and canola oil. Polyunsaturated fats include most other plant oils, including safflower, soybean, corn, sunflower, sesame, and cottonseed oil, as well as fish, walnuts, hazelnuts, pecans, almonds, and peanuts. Unsaturated fat is the kind you should eat because:

• It's a great energy source;

• It contains those aforementioned essential fatty acids;

• It actually *lowers* blood cholesterol levels.

In terms of your heart's health, the amount of trans fat and saturated fat you consume is more important than the total amount of fat in your diet. Health experts recommend substituting healthy unsaturated fats (monounsaturated and polyunsaturated) for the bad kind—for example, using natural vegetable oils in cooking.

How Much Fat Should You Eat?

Most health experts recommend limiting fat to no more than 30 percent of total daily calories, though some think 20 percent is preferable, with less than 10 percent of calories from saturated fat. And when you're trying to lose weight, you may want to limit your fat intake to 20 or 25 percent of calories.

You can figure out your daily fat intake by reading nutrition labels on the foods you use. (See chapter 5 for more on using food labels to figure out fat content.) These labels are based on a 2,000-calorie diet; so if you eat 2,000 calories a day, you'd figure:

Calories from fat should be no more than 600
 (2,000 × 0.30 = 600)
or no more than about 67 grams fat
 (600 calories divided by 9 calories per gram of fat = 67).

SMART SOURCES

These fat-counter guides are handy reference sources:

American Heart Association Fat and Cholesterol Counter
American Heart Association

Fat Counter
Annette Natow and JoAnn Heslin

If you're aiming for 20 percent of your calories from fat, that would come out to 400 calories, or no more than about 44 grams of fat. Remember, that's for a 2,000-calorie diet; when you're on a lower-calorie diet, you can easily adjust the numbers accordingly.

Recommended Upper Limits of Total Fat and Saturated Fat Intake at Different Calorie Levels

1,200   Total fat, 40 grams; saturated fat, 16 grams

1,600   Total fat, 53 grams; saturated fat, 18 grams

2,000   Total fat, 65 grams; saturated fat, 20 grams

2,500   Total fat, 80 grams; saturated fat, 25 grams

Why Less Fat Isn't Always Better

Many health experts worry about diets in which much less than 30 percent of calories come from fats, since lower-fat diets can reduce blood levels of heart-protecting HDLs (high-density lipoproteins) and raise heart-damaging triglycerides. And extremely-low-fat diets may interfere with the intake of essential nutrients in children, pregnant women, and the elderly.

Another problem is that people on very-low-fat diets often replace fats with carbohydrates in the form of sugars and refined starches, which can increase your coronary risk if you're inactive—and can actually make you pack on pounds instead of shedding them.

The Perils of Cholesterol

Cholesterol is a fatlike substance manufactured by your body and also found in high-saturated-fat animal foods such as:

• Egg yolks;

• Meat, poultry, and fish;

• High-fat milk products.

Cholesterol is essential for various physical functions: It's an important part of cell membranes and a building block for important hormones. However, your body makes at least enough cholesterol to fulfill these functions; some people manufacture more than they need and have naturally elevated blood-cholesterol levels. Excess cholesterol, whether manufactured by your body or provided by a diet high in saturated fat and cholesterol, contributes to the development of atherosclerosis, in which the arteries narrow and reduce blood circulation. This can lead to heart attack or stroke.

That's why it's wise to keep an eye on your cholesterol level (your doctor can measure it for you and let you know if it's too high) and take steps to keep it in check. That doesn't mean you need to eliminate all high-cholesterol foods from your diet; many of them are also high in essential nutrients. But most people can keep cholesterol under control by getting plenty of exercise and eating a diet rich in whole grains, fruits, and vegetables.

In fact, you are better off watching out for saturated fats, which are found in many of the same foods—but not all the same foods. Saturated fats

SMART MONEY

"The fat-free craze has become so widespread that Americans have actually succeeded, in the past decade, in cutting their average fat intake from 36 percent to 34 percent," writes Laura Fraser in *Losing It: America's Obsession with Weight and the Industry That Feeds on It.*

Despite this success, notes Fraser, in this same period the average American has become eight pounds heavier. "It's a paradox: we're eating less fat and getting fatter."

raise cholesterol levels more than does dietary cholesterol. Translation: Eating shrimp, which are high in cholesterol but contain unsaturated fat, is better for you than eating "cholesterol-free" cookies, which are likely to be laden with saturated or hydrogenated fat.

Confused? The simple solution is to check nutrition labels for saturated fat and simply ignore those "cholesterol-free" claims. (See chapter 6 for more on reading nutrition labels.)

The Good and Bad News about Reduced-Fat Foods

It's true that by limiting fat, you're likely to lower your calories as well—but beware! The wide availability and consumption of reduced-fat and fat-free foods such as cookies and other baked goods would seem to be good news for the weight-conscious, but it's not necessarily so.

Why? Well, it seems that the words "fat free" or "reduced fat" on, say, a bag of cookies trigger some sort of free-for-all mentality in many people, encouraging them to eat twice as much as they otherwise would. Never mind that fat-free or reduced-fat items may contain almost or as many calories as, if not more than, their fattier relatives.

In a recent study, a group of women were fed yogurt that was labeled either "high-fat" or "low-fat"—although in fact all the yogurt was the same. The women then ate lunch. The women who had the so-called low-fat yogurt ate more lunch than did the group who ate the so-called high-fat yogurt. Researchers concluded that the study subjects regarded the low-fat label as a "license to overeat."

When companies make low-fat foods, they often replace fat with sugar so the food will still taste good. Replacing fat with sugar, however, also increases appetite. And because the fat in food gives you a satisfied feeling of fullness, its absence may lead you to eat more to compensate.

Of course, it's a very good thing, healthwise, to cut down on your fat intake, but as far as weight loss goes, you still need to watch your overall calorie intake, and eating a whole bag of anything is not going to speed you on your way to sylph-hood. And it's damaging not only to your poundage but also to your long-term mind-set—learning to eat

Fat Substitutes: Answer to Weight-Loss Prayers?

Fat substitutes are designed to provide all the satisfying qualities of fat—flavor, texture, and mouth feel—without the calories, saturated fat, and cholesterol. With 0 to 4 calories per gram, products such as Olestra are now being used to make typically high-fat foods such as potato chips, crackers, and other snacks, leading many to hope for a future of limitless, guilt-free snacking.

How do they work? Olestra, for example, provides no calories and no fat, because it is indigestible—it was created in a form that can't be absorbed by the body. Because of this, it can cause intestinal cramps and other side effects and, like other such fat substitutes, inhibits the absorption of some vitamins. For this reason, health experts worry about a future in which fat substitutes may become a major part of American diets.

But can they help you lose weight? That's not yet clear. In one study, a group of men were given a breakfast of regular fat-containing foods, and another group was given Olestra-containing foods. Those who ate the Olestra-containing foods made up their usual daily caloric intake by eating more carbohydrate-containing foods. This indicates that foods containing fat substitutes, like other fat-reduced products, may help reduce fat intake but not total calories.

Recommended Daily Protein Intake

Age	Weight	Protein Needed
Children		
1 to 3 yrs.	29 lbs.	16 g.
4 to 6 yrs.	44 lbs.	24 g.
7 to 10 yrs.	62 lbs.	28 g.
Men and boys		
11 to 14 yrs.	99 lbs.	45 g.
15 to 18 yrs.	145 lbs.	59 g.
19 to 24 yrs.	160 lbs.	59 g.
25 or older	174 lbs.	63 g.
Women and girls		
11 to 14 yrs.	101 lbs.	46 g.
15 to 18 yrs.	120 lbs.	44 g.
19 to 24 yrs.	128 lbs.	46 g.
25 or older	138 lbs.	50 g.
Pregnant women		60 g.
Nursing mothers		
First 6 months		65 g.
Second 6 months		63 g.

Source: National Academy of Sciences

in moderation is a big part of the weight-loss equation, and a "fat-free" label does not constitute an exception to the rule.

The best advice: Look at the Nutrition Facts panel on food labels (discussed in chapter 6) to compare calories and other nutrition information between fat-reduced and regular-fat foods. Don't kid yourself.

Protein Facts

Protein provides your body with nine essential amino acids, chemical compounds that serve as the building blocks, repairers, and regenerators of muscle and tissue, necessary for a strong, muscular body. Your body contains anywhere from ten thousand to fifty thousand kinds of protein; everything from hair to skin to blood to enzymes and hormones is made of the stuff. But beware of those who tell you you can't get enough protein in your diet: Consuming more than your body needs is not only unnecessary but potentially harmful.

True, it's essential to consume protein daily because your body cannot store it the way it stores fats. But it's pretty easy to get enough in a basic, well-balanced diet; in fact, most Americans consume more than enough.

How Much Do You Need?

Nutritionists generally warn against eating more than the Recommended Daily Allowance because many protein-rich foods are high in fat, and high-protein diets are hard on your kidneys and may damage them. And eating a disproportionate amount of protein in an attempt to hasten weight loss can wreak havoc on your metabolism.

The RDA for women over twenty-five is 50 grams, an amount that's easy to consume even when trying to lose weight. For men it's 63 grams.

Complete versus Incomplete Proteins, and Where to Find Them

Complete proteins (also known as animal proteins) contain all the amino acids you need, in the amounts you need to stay healthy. They are found in animal foods such as:

• Eggs;

• Meat;

• Fish;

• Poultry;

• Milk and other dairy products.

Incomplete proteins (also known as vegetable proteins) lack one or more essential amino acids.

F.Y.I.

The Zone, a hugely popular high-protein diet developed by biochemist Barry Sears, is based on the premise that consuming 40 percent carbohydrate (rather than the generally recommended 60 percent), 30 percent protein, and 30 percent fat at every meal will reduce body fat by affecting the body's hormonal systems. Zone dieters are not allowed such foods as pasta, breakfast cereal, bread, bananas, and other high-carbohydrate foods. Does it work? Well, yes, it will probably help you lose weight, but health experts agree it's highly likely that low-calorie content rather than specific food combinations are responsible.

SMART SOURCES

You'll find lots of great vegetarian menus and healthy eating tips in these tomes:

Amazing Grains: Creating Vegetarian Main Dishes with Whole Grains Joanne Saltzman; Jay Harlow (ed.)

American Wholefoods Cuisine: 1,300 Meatless, Wholesome Recipes from Short Order to Gourmet Nikki and David Goldbeck

The New Laurel's Kitchen: A Handbook for Vegetarian Cooking Laurel Robertson, Carol Flinders, and Brian Ruppenthal

The following plant foods are good sources of incomplete protein:

• Legumes, including peanuts, dried beans, peas, and soybeans;

• Grains, especially whole grains;

• Potatoes.

The Vegetarian Way: Combining Proteins

Two incomplete proteins can be combined to make a complete protein—an important trick to learn if you're a vegetarian or simply limit your consumption of animal foods. It happens like this: When you eat a food that lacks a specific amino acid with another food that supplies the missing amino acid, you end up with a high-quality protein.

Now, you don't have to know the amino acid composition of every food you eat in order to make sure you're getting complete proteins, and you don't need to eat complete proteins at every meal. But you do need to educate yourself about the right foods to eat to ensure adequate nutrition. Some of the classics include:

• Rice and beans;

• Soup and bread;

• A peanut butter sandwich.

Check the vegetarian cookbook section at your local bookstore or library for an abundance of other great ideas. And find out more about smart vegetarian eating in chapter 5.

What about High-Protein Diets?

Diets that advocate eating twice as much protein as carbohydrates come in and go out of style like miniskirts. There's a reason for their popularity: In the short run they'll help you lose weight, and fast. But in the long run they're very bad news.

Here's how they work: When you stop eating much in the way of carbohydrates, your body immediately loses water, which is reflected as weight loss on the scale. You also lose an essential source of energy, glucose, which is supplied by carbohydrates. Without sufficient glucose, your body turns to its fat stores for energy.

This may sound like a promising weight-loss scenario; in fact, it's anything but. Eventually your body goes into ketosis, a food-deprived mode in which your metabolism slows down and your body no longer burns fat. Not only is this very unhealthy, but it makes losing more weight harder and harder, and it can screw up your metabolism for life.

As usual, the shortcut to weight loss doesn't pay off.

Carbohydrate Facts

Carbohydrates are sugars and starches that provide most of your body fuel and keep your central nervous system, and thus your brain, in working

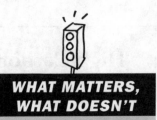

WHAT MATTERS, WHAT DOESN'T

What Matters

• Making sure you include protein in your diet every day.

• Avoiding protein overload, which can make your body sick.

What Doesn't

• Eating animal foods to get protein; you can get all you need by combining plant foods.

High-Carbohydrate Lows

Some people don't do well on high-carbohydrate diets, especially those high in processed carbohydrates—white rice, white flour, and products made from them. If you find yourself tired and draggy and unable to shed pounds even after cutting calories, you may need to trim your carbohydrate intake (and increase your fat somewhat).

order. In other words, they're crucial. That's why most nutrition experts recommend getting about 60 percent of your daily calories from carbohydrates.

When carbohydrates enter your body, they break down into a simple sugar called glucose. Glucose enters your bloodstream and supplies you with physical and mental energy; it is also stored as glycogen—a readily available form of glucose—in the liver and muscle tissue, to provide energy reserves. Because your body constantly needs its glycogen stores replenished—particularly if you are active—carbohydrate calories are more likely to be used as glycogen than converted to fat. This is a good thing, weight-loss–wise.

Simple versus Complex

Two types of carbohydrates—simple and complex—provide fuel to your body. Simple carbohydrates are easily converted to glucose and are quickly absorbed into your blood, giving you a jolt of energy. They're found in:

• Sugar (both white and brown);

• Other sweeteners, such as maple syrup, corn syrup, molasses, and honey;

• Sweet desserts such as cookies and cakes;

• Candy bars;

• Fruit and fruit juices;

• Cola and other sodas.

Complex carbohydrates, on the other hand, are made up of hundreds or thousands of glucose molecules and break down more slowly, especially if the foods that contain them also contain fiber. This means complex carbohydrates are an excellent source of slow-burning energy, the kind that's fueled many a marathon runner. Sources include:

• Pasta, rice, bread, cereal, flour, and other grains;

• Potatoes and other root vegetables;

• Dried peas and beans;

• Starchy vegetables such as winter squash and corn.

From a glance at these two lists, you can figure out that complex carbohydrates are, overall, the better category for the scale-conscious. No empty calories—the kind that are high in sugar or fat, low in nutrients—are to be found here. And many complex carbohydrates provide fiber, which not only makes for longer-lasting energy but also fills you up so you want to eat less. (For more on the benefits of fiber, see chapter 4.)

However, it's not that black and white. Some simple carbohydrates, such as fruit and fruit juices,

The Lowdown on Sugar Substitutes

Sugar substitutes such as sorbitol, saccharine, and aspartame can help cut calories, no question. But they probably won't make a significant dent in your total calorie tally. And because there's some controversy about their safety, you're best off not consuming massive quantities.

However, there's good news on the sweet front: An herb called stevia, which has long been used abroad, is now becoming available in the United States. One teaspoon is as sweet as three cups of sugar but contains only eight calories. Now sold as a dietary supplement, it has yet to be reviewed for safety by the FDA, but numerous studies have indicated it's a safe, natural option.

are nutritional dynamos, and some complex carbohydrates, such as white flour and white rice, which are high in processed carbohydrates, are fairly low on the nutrient scale.

Good and Not-So-Good Sugars

Lots of people think of sugar as an unnecessary, albeit good-tasting, addition to food—the stuff you spoon out of a bowl at breakfast. But sugar is produced by the body during carbohydrate breakdown, and it also occurs naturally in many nutritious foods such as milk, fruits, vegetables, cereals, breads, and grains.

So even if you wanted to, you probably couldn't eliminate all sugars from your diet. Nor should you try. Sugar, despite its iffy reputation, is not bad for you, and avoiding sugars alone will not make you lose weight. And despite much suspicion to the contrary, scientific evidence indicates that diets high in sugars do not cause hyperactivity or diabetes.

However, sugar and many sugary foods, such as sodas, cookies, and other snacks, do provide lots of calories and very little or no nutrition. Don't kid yourself that honey or brown sugar is a more healthful, less-caloric substitute for regular sugar; it all comes down to the same thing. And they definitely promote tooth decay.

To lose weight, you should cut down on empty calories in any form, including sugar-coated. But as far as your health is concerned, a little sprinkle of sugar now and then won't hurt you.

THE BOTTOM LINE

Understanding the building blocks of nutrition enables you to choose your own sensible eating plan without following anyone else's rigid prescriptions or falling into any gimmicky weight-loss traps. When you learn what your body needs and why, eating right becomes the smart, easy choice.

Non-caloric Nutrients

Fat, protein, and carbohydrates may have a higher profile among the weight-conscious, but noncaloric nutrients—including vitamins, minerals, fiber, and water—are just as essential to a healthy diet. And although these substances themselves don't contain calories, you're best off eating them in caloric containers; that is, instead of popping a pill, try to get your fill from the foods you eat.

Vitamins and Minerals

Contrary to popular myth, vitamins and minerals do not provide energy. What they do is regulate biochemical reactions in your body. Translation: They perform essential functions that enable you to live.

Vital Vitamins

There are thirteen known vitamins—organic compounds that are required to keep the body healthy and free of disease. Some, such as A and D, are fat-soluble and can damage the liver if consumed in excess amounts; others, such as C, are water-soluble, and excess amounts will be flushed out of the body. The following section lists those you need and the best food sources for each. (Chapter 5 has more information on top nutritious food choices.)

Vitamins

Vitamin: A

Function: Growth and tissue repair, healthy skin, and night and color vision; its precursor, beta-carotene, is an antioxidant.

Found in: Carrots, sweet potatoes, tomatoes, and other red, yellow, and orange fruits and vegetables; also leafy green vegetables.

Recommended Dietary Allowance: 5,000 IUs (International Units)

Vitamin: B_1 (Thiamin)

Function: Converts carbohydrates into energy; regulates function of the heart, muscles, nerves, and digestive system.

Found in: Legumes, nuts, meat, oatmeal, and enriched cereals and bread.

Recommended Dietary Allowance: 1.5 milligrams

Vitamin: B_2 (Riboflavin)

Function: Growth, energy production, maintaining immune system and healthy skin and mucous membranes.

Found in: Dairy products, meat, enriched cereals, almonds.

Recommended Dietary Allowance: 1.7 milligrams

SMART DEFINITION

Antioxidants
Antioxidants are chemicals, including vitamins C and E and beta-carotene (which converts to vitamin A in the body), that may be a major force in preventing cancer. They are believed to destroy unstable molecules, known as free radicals, that may help form cancers and cataracts as well as accelerate aging. And antioxidants may also help prevent heart disease by preventing arterial plaque buildup.

Vitamin: B_3 (Niacin)

Function: Energy production, healthy digestive and reproductive systems, healthy skin, mood regulation.

Found in: Legumes, nuts, meat, poultry, seafood, leafy green vegetables, enriched cereals.

Recommended Dietary Allowance: 20 milligrams

Vitamin: B_6 (Pyridoxine)

Function: Growth, energy production, red-blood-cell production; may help treat symptoms of PMS.

Found in: Meat, poultry, seafood, legumes, leafy green vegetables, bananas, enriched cereals.

Recommended Dietary Allowance: 2.0 milligrams

Vitamin: B_{12} (Cobalamin)

Function: Energy production, red-blood-cell production, mental health; long-term deficiency is associated with Alzheimer's disease.

Found in: Dairy products, meat, poultry, seafood, mushrooms, tempeh.

Recommended Dietary Allowance: 6.0 micrograms

Vitamin: B_7 (Biotin)

Function: Energy production, protein and fat metabolism.

Found in: Egg yolks; also found in small amounts in other foods.

Recommended Dietary Allowance: 0.3 milligram

Vitamin: B_9 (Folic acid)

Function: Energy production, red-blood-cell production, growth and development; deficiency may cause birth defects.

Found in: Legumes, whole grains, leafy green vegetables, meat, seafood.

Recommended Dietary Allowance: 400 micrograms

Vitamin: B_5 (Pantothenic acid)

Function: Protein, fat, and carbohydrate metabolism; growth.

Found in: Legumes, whole grains, meat, poultry, seafood.

Recommended Dietary Allowance: 10 milligrams

Vitamin: C

Function: Growth, bone and tooth formation, iron absorption, healing, disease resistance; antioxidant.

Found in: Citrus fruit, berries, tomatoes, cauliflower, peppers, leafy green vegetables.

Recommended Dietary Allowance: 60 milligrams

Vitamin: D

Function: Growth; bone, tooth, and nail formation; part of calcium absorption system.

Found in: Fortified milk and milk products, fatty fish; the body also manufactures vitamin D when sunlight falls on the skin.

Recommended Dietary Allowance: 400 IUs (International Units)

Vitamin: E

Function: Protects nerves and cell membranes; joint and ligament health; antioxidant.

Found in: Avocado, broccoli, asparagus, sunflower seeds, vegetable oils.

Recommended Dietary Allowance: 30 IUs (International Units)

Vitamin: K

Function: Bone formation, blood clotting.

Found in: Dairy products, leafy green vegetables, broccoli.

Recommended Dietary Allowance: None established

Do You Need a Supplement?

According to the American Medical Association, if you're a healthy adult who's not pregnant or breast-feeding, you don't require supplements, as long as you eat a well-balanced diet made up of all the major food groups.

But despite your best intentions, you may come up short. Hectic schedules, meals on the run, and low-calorie diets can all wreak havoc on your nutritional good intentions. So there's nothing wrong with taking a vitamin/mineral supplement as a sort of insurance policy. Women, in particular, have trouble getting enough bone-saving calcium in their diet, so they're well advised to take a daily calcium supplement.

But don't think a supplement can take the place of smart eating and "fix" long-term deficiencies in your diet. Scientists still aren't sure whether your body uses the vitamins and minerals in supplements the same way it uses those found in foods. And there's increasing evidence that essential nutrients called phytochemicals, which are found in foods from green plants, have health-protective powers not found in any pill.

If you do choose a vitamin/mineral supplement, the Food and Nutrition Board of the National Research Council recommends avoiding supplements that exceed 100 percent of the RDA. Megadoses of vitamins A, D, and E, and many minerals, can serious harm your vital organs, and they can also interfere with the absorption of other nutrients.

Vital Minerals

Like vitamins, minerals are vital to keep energy flowing through our bodies. They are found in enzymes and hormones, and they are used to break down carbohydrates and fats. There are more than

SMART DEFINITION

Phytochemicals
Compounds known as "functional foods"—neither vitamins nor minerals—that occur naturally in fruits and vegetables; researchers believe they have potential as cancer-fighting agents.

SMART DEFINITION

Chelated minerals
Absorption is increased if the mineral is chelated, which means the mineral is bound with a benign salt, such as citrate, picolinate, gluconate, or aspartate. This process, which changes the electrical charge, is why, for example, a label will read "magnesium citrate" instead of magnesium.

three dozen known dietary minerals, but only nineteen are known to be essential for our health. Most of these are needed only in trace amounts, but they're all needed nonetheless. The section below lists some of the most common minerals, why you need them, and the best places to find them.

Minerals

Mineral: Calcium

Function: Bone formation and strength; too little calcium leaves women at risk for osteoporosis.

Found in: Milk and other dairy products, sardines (with bones), leafy green vegetables, dried fruit, nuts, whole wheat bread.

Recommended Dietary Allowance: 1 gram

Mineral: Copper

Function: Maintains enzyme system, essential for red-blood-cell formation.

Found in: Red meat, oysters, nuts, olive oil.

Recommended Dietary Allowance: 2.0 milligrams

Mineral: Iodine

Function: Maintains function of thyroid gland and thyroid hormones.

Found in: Saltwater fish, iodized salt.

Recommended Dietary Allowance: 150 micrograms

Mineral: Iron

Function: Transports oxygen to the cells; too little can cause anemia, fatigue, and depression.

Found in: Red meat, poultry, shellfish, legumes, leafy green vegetables, dried fruit, molasses.

Recommended Dietary Allowance: 18 milligrams

Mineral: Manganese

Function: Bone formation, energy production, protein metabolism.

Found in: Whole grain cereals, nuts, tea.

Recommended Dietary Allowance: None established

Mineral: Phosphorus

Function: Maintains muscle and nerve function.

Found in: Almost all foods; calcium-rich foods are the best source.

Recommended Dietary Allowance: 1 gram

Mineral: Potassium

Function: Balances body fluids, maintains nervous system.

Found in: Fruit (especially bananas), dried fruit, vegetables, legumes, milk.

Recommended Dietary Allowance: 3,500 milligrams

F.Y.I.

Check out some of the new calcium-rich foods at the supermarket. Many breakfast cereals (hot and cold) and breads now have extra calcium. And the favorite breakfast drink, orange juice, is now also calcium-fortified. There's even calcium-enriched beer.

Mineral: Selenium

Function: Antioxidant; helps control cholesterol; helps protect the body from cancer.

Found in: Meat, seafood, grains, nuts (especially Brazil nuts).

Recommended Dietary Allowance: None established

Mineral: Sodium

Function: Regulates body fluids, muscle and nerve function.

Found in: Almost all foods.

Recommended Dietary Allowance: 2,400 milligrams

Mineral: Zinc

Function: Growth, healing, natural resistance, reproduction, appetite, and taste.

Found in: Meat, poultry, shellfish, eggs, legumes, garlic, ginger root, wheat germ, almonds.

Recommended Dietary Allowance: 15 milligrams

Spotlight on Calcium

This nutrient deserves singling out because it's the one most are likely to stint on when watching calories. Getting enough calcium is essential, for maintaining a healthy body now and for staving off the future risk of osteoporosis, the brittle-bone disease that affects many older women.

Although calcium is found in a wide variety of foods, it can be tricky to get enough because your body can't utilize it unless it has a sufficient amount of other nutrients, such as phosphorus and magnesium, and hormones, such as estrogen. And any of the following can interfere with its absorption:

• Consuming caffeine (more than two cups of coffee a day) or soda;

• Smoking;

• Eating large amounts of protein;

• Eating lots of salty foods.

If you add a low-calorie diet to this mix, you're more than likely to be missing out on what you need.

The RDA for premenopausal women is 800 milligrams a day, but the National Institutes of Health advocates an optimal intake of 1,000 milligrams, and 1,500 if you're pregnant or postmenopausal (and not on hormone replacement therapy).

The best bet is to eat a diet high in calcium-rich foods and take a calcium supplement to be sure you're getting all you need. There are many low-fat, high-nutrition choices:

• Vegetables such as kale and broccoli;

• Low-fat yogurt and skim milk;

• Mineral water, which contains calcium.

For more calcium-rich sources, see chapter 5.

Another important factor is exercise: Lots of

walking, biking, weight-training, and other forms of weight-bearing exercise are great for your bones. And be sure to get out in the sunlight whenever you can—exposure to the sun makes your body produce vitamin D, which helps you absorb calcium.

Good and Bad Sodium

There's lots of confusion about sodium and salt. On the one hand, sodium is one of the minerals essential to your body's health. On the other hand, salt (sodium chloride) isn't good for you—or is it?

Sodium is the main nonwater component of the body's extracellular fluids and helps carry nutrients into the cells; it also helps regulate blood pressure. However, the amount of sodium the body needs is minimal.

As for salt, not all scientists agree it's a bad thing. Most believe that if you don't have high blood pressure, you needn't worry about salting your baked potato. But if you are at risk for hypertension, you need to keep your salt intake to a strict minimum; hypertension can lead in turn to heart attack, kidney disease, and stroke. And some health experts also warn that excess salt intake makes your kidneys work too hard to get rid of the excess, resulting in a loss of calcium.

Then, too, there's the matter of bloat. Cutting down on your salt intake can really help if you tend to retain water.

One teaspoon of salt provides about 2,300 milligrams of sodium, so it's easy to consume more than the 2,400 or so milligrams generally recommended for healthy people. Some 75 percent of the sodium Americans consume comes from processed foods—bread, cheese, canned foods, and more. So pushing away the salt shaker at home or at a restaurant won't help much.

To reduce your salt intake, try the following:

• Become alert to hidden sources of salt in your diet by reading nutrition labels when you shop (see chapter 6).

• Seek out lower-sodium alternatives to your favorite foods; often they taste just as good, or better.

• If you need to add salt when cooking, do it at the end; you're likely to add much less.

• Cut down gradually; you may find yourself losing your taste for salty foods.

When you do eat salty foods, increase your potassium intake by eating lots of fresh fruits and vegetables: Potassium may help reduce blood pressure.

Two Other Essentials: Fiber and Water

Vital to good health, fiber and water are also low-key stars in any smart weight-loss plan. Not only do they both perform essential functions in your body, but they also help control your appetite and give you a satisfied "full" feeling—all at a low- or no-calorie price.

F.Y.I.

Recent research from the USDA's Human Nutrition Research Center indicates that if you double your daily fiber intake from an average of 18 grams to 36 grams, you can reduce the absorption of fat and protein from other foods by about 130 calories a day. In one year that adds up to thirteen pounds of weight loss!

Fiber Facts

The carbohydrate fiber contains no calories or nutrients (though it comes packaged in foods that contain them), and it passes through your body in undigested form. That may not sound very promising, healthwise, but in fact eating fiber is one of the best things you can do for your body.

Fiber has been found to aid digestion and prevent constipation, as well as help ward off hemorrhoids, and it's strongly suspected of lowering the risk for heart disease and some cancers. Therefore the National Cancer Institute and the American Dietetic Association recommend that Americans consume lots of it: 20 to 35 grams of fiber a day. Somewhere in the middle of that range is a good place to start; too much can lead to bloating and diarrhea. And remember, the more fiber you eat, the more water you should drink as well, to keep all that roughage moving through your body.

Where to get it? Fiber's found in many of the same healthy foods you should be eating if you're watching your weight and fat intake:

• Fruits and vegetables;

• Legumes;

• Whole-grain breads;

• Oatmeal;

• Bran.

For more high-fiber food choices, see chapter 5.

Water Wisdom

A few years back, everyone suddenly started traipsing around with water bottles strapped to their side, poking out of a backpack, or glued to their lips. Water had turned into a fashion statement. But beneath the trend lies some basic, timeless common sense. Water—be it the expensive designer brands or plain old filtered tap water—is essential to your body, as essential as the air you breathe. It's always your best liquid bet, particularly when you're trying to shed pounds. Yet despite the ubiquitous water bottles, many people still drink far less fluid than they should.

Here's what water does for your health:

• Keeps your body hydrated;

• Aids digestion and metabolism;

• Helps flush out waste and toxins.

And here's what water does for your weight-loss efforts:

• Helps fill you up—without calories;

• Helps suppress your appetite; in fact, it's easy to confuse hunger and thirst; the next time you think you're hungry, try drinking a glass of water and see if your hunger abates;

• When used in place of other liquids, it helps you cut back on calories easily and painlessly.

How Much Do You Need?

You must constantly replenish your body's supply of water; you lose at least ten cups a day through breathing, perspiration, evaporation, and excretion. You can replenish a certain amount of water by drinking other liquids and eating fruits and vegetables, but you should also try to drink a minimum of sixty-four ounces of water (at least eight cups) a day. It's especially wise to drink a glass before and after a workout to prevent dehydration.

Here's a good way to tell if you're drinking enough water and other fluids: Check the color of your urine. If it's medium to dark yellow you need to drink more.

THE BOTTOM LINE

When you're trying to lose weight, it's easy to focus on what you shouldn't eat and forget about what you *should* and *must* eat in order to stay healthy. To both look and feel your best, tallying your vitamin, mineral, fiber, and water intake is as important as counting fat grams.

CHAPTER 5

The Best Foods

THE KEYS

• The USDA Food Guide Pyramid is designed to keep the public in good health, but it is also appropriate for weight loss.

• Grains are a sure-fire bet for healthful, satisfying weight loss and to get in disease-fighting nutrients.

• Fruits and vegetables are your most nutritious fare and will go a long way to aiding you in your weight-loss efforts.

• Dairy foods are calcium-rich and an important part of a nutritional plan, but they need not be calorie-dense and loaded with fat.

• Proteins are nutrient-packed, and there is a a wide range of protein sources to choose from, whether you are carnivore or vegetarian.

A smart weight-loss strategy means thinking in terms of *adding* to your diet rather than taking away. Eating a wide variety of good-for-you foods will not only put you in fighting trim but is guaranteed to banish same-old same-old diet malaise. But how do you know which foods to choose, and how much to eat? The easiest and best way to start is with some guidance from the experts.

The Food Guide Pyramid

If you've ever examined the U.S. Department of Agriculture's Food Guide Pyramid, you may have come away with two impressions:

1. You can't be bothered memorizing some chart that's probably aimed at fifth graders; it's not relevant to your lifestyle.

2. It may be healthy, but you'd be twice as fat if you ate all that.

Well, you're right—and wrong.

The Food Guide Pyramid wasn't designed for weight loss, but it definitely was designed with good health and nutrition in mind. And you know the connection between those three elements.

True to its name, the pyramid is best used as a guide, not a set of immutable rules. There's no need to hang a giant pyramid chart in your kitchen and check off your daily servings from each food group, but reviewing the basics really can help you keep your yen for, say, starchy foods in check by reminding you of the need for balance.

The pyramid is useful because it enables you to think in terms of servings rather than calories. For many people, this is a much easier and more pleasant way to live. Not only is counting calories exceedingly dull, but it is also an unnatural, restrictive way of eating, one that you're more than likely to rebel against sooner or later.

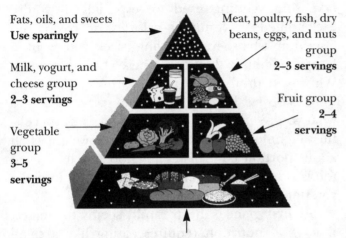

Fats, oils, and sweets
Use sparingly

Meat, poultry, fish, dry beans, eggs, and nuts group
2–3 servings

Milk, yogurt, and cheese group
2–3 servings

Fruit group
2–4 servings

Vegetable group
3–5 servings

Bread, cereal, rice, and pasta group **6–11 servings**

Instead of the traditional four food groups, the pyramid has six, starting at the bottom with those foods you should eat most often:

• Choose most of your calories from foods in the bread, cereal, rice, and pasta group (six to eleven servings), the vegetable group (three to five servings), and the fruit group (two to four servings).

• Eat moderate amounts of foods from the milk, yogurt, and cheese group (two to three servings) and the meat, poultry, fish, dry beans, eggs, and nuts group (two to three servings).

• Limit foods in the fats, oils, and sweets group (consume sparingly).

Serving Sizes

Thinking about eating in terms of servings may take some getting used to, especially if you're accustomed to counting calories or paying no attention whatsoever. Serving sizes represent a happy medium between these two extremes. When you think in terms of portions, you don't have to obsess, but you do have to pay attention to what you're eating—a central tenet of any successful weight-loss plan. At heart, losing weight is all about portion control. Eating too much of even foods that are good for you is not going to make you slender.

At first glance, the pyramid seems to suggest that good nutrition requires eating like a small elephant. But the servings aren't as big as you might imagine: For example, one serving of pasta is half a cup; most people eat two or more servings at a sitting. If you're carrying around excess poundage, you've probably been eating way more than the recommended amounts.

However, the whole point of the pyramid is flexibility, so if you find you're eating more than you want or you're not losing weight, cut back on the serving sizes—but not on any one food group.

How Many Servings Should You Eat?

You'll notice a range of servings for each food group. The smaller number is for people who aim to lose weight gradually by consuming about 1,500 to 1,600 calories a day (about right for a five-foot, four-inch moderately active adult woman; your calorie level may need adjustment depending on height, weight, and current activity level). The larger number is for those who want to consume about 2,800 calories a day, which is probably not you unless you are extremely active. (Refer to chapter 2 for more on target calorie goal.)

Some foods fit into more than one category. Starchy vegetables—for example, potatoes, sweet potatoes, and corn—can be counted as either grains or vegetables, and dry beans, peas, and lentils are in the meat group but can be counted as servings of vegetables instead. These crossover foods can be counted as servings from either one or the other group, but not both.

Don't think that by eating the same few foods from each group you're covering all the bases. It's important to choose a variety of foods within each group to be sure you're getting a wider range of nutrients. For example, some vegetables and fruits are good sources of vitamin A or C, while others are high in folic acid; still others are good sources of calcium or iron. Plus variety is the key to staving off dietary boredom.

You may be one of those people who bridle at the very notion of eating according to food groups and serving sizes, but the food pyramid is actually more about choices than limitations. Make the most of it by trying a wide range of foods in each group, and you'll never feel like you're living behind bars.

How Big Is a Serving?

Food Group	Serving Size
Bread, cereal, rice, and pasta	1 slice bread (preferably whole grain); ½ English muffin or bagel; 1 small corn tortilla; 5 or 6 small crackers; 1 ounce ready-to-eat cereal; ½ cup cooked cereal, rice, or pasta; ¼ cup corn, potatoes, legumes, or other starchy vegetable.
Vegetable	1 cup raw, leafy vegetables; ½ cup cooked or chopped raw vegetables; ¾ cup vegetable juice.
Fruit	1 medium fresh fruit (e.g., apple, banana, or orange); 1 cup berries; ½ grapefruit; ½ cup chopped, cooked, or canned fruit; ¾ cup fruit juice; 2 tablespoons raisins; 7 dried apricot halves; 10 grapes; 10 cherries.
Milk, yogurt, and cheese	8 ounces low- or nonfat milk or yogurt; 1½ ounces natural cheese; ½ cup skim-milk ricotta; 8 ounces low-fat and calcium-fortified soy milk.
Meat, poultry, fish, dry beans, eggs, and nuts	2 to 3 ounces cooked, lean meat, chicken, fish, veal, or pork (less than 5 grams of fat per ounce). Other foods that count as 1 ounce meat: ½ cup cooked dry beans, peas, or lentils; 1 egg; 2 table-spoons peanut butter (preferably the reduced-fat kind, containing 2 grams of fat per serving); ⅓ cup nuts.

Source: United States Department of Agriculture

The table below shows how many servings of each major food group can be included at different calorie levels.

1,600 calories

For many sedentary women and some older adults

Bread Group . . . . 6 servings

Fruit Group . . . . 2 servings

Vegetable Group . . . . 3 servings

Milk Group. . . . . 2 to 3 servings

Meat Group. . . . . 5 ounces

2,200 calories*

For most children, teenage girls, active women, and many sedentary men

Bread Group . . . . 9 servings

Fruit Group . . . . 3 servings

Vegetable Group . . . . 4 servings

Milk Group. . . . . 2 to 3 servings**

Meat Group. . . . . 6 ounces

* Pregnant or breast-feeding women need more calories.

**Pregnant or breast-feeding women, as well as teenagers and young adults to age twenty-four, need 3 servings.

SMART MONEY

"You can't just change your lifestyle all at once," says Weight Watchers psychologist Ronna Kabatznick. "That would be like trying to get your Ph.D. in a week. People who are successful meet many small, gradual goals that add up to a total lifestyle change."

SMART SOURCES

Here are two prime sources of nutrition information:

International Food
    Information Council
1100 Connecticut Ave.
    NW, Suite 430
Washington, DC 20036
202-296-6540
http://www.ificinfo.
health.org

United States Depart-
    ment of Agriculture
    Center for Nutrition
    Policy and Promotion
1120 20th St. NW,
Suite 200
Washington, DC 20036
202-418-2312
http://www.usda.gov/
fcs/cnpp

2,800 calories

For teenage boys, active men, and some very active women

Bread Group . . . . 11 servings

Fruit Group . . . . 4 servings

Vegetable Group . . . . 5 servings

Milk Group. . . . . 2 to 3 servings

Meat Group. . . . . 7 ounces

Some things to remember when you put the Food Guide Pyramid to use:

• Even when you're trying to lose weight and consume fewer calories, you should still eat from all the food groups, but in smaller amounts. For example, women can start by eating the suggested servings for a 1,600-calorie diet; if you find you aren't losing weight, simply reduce the number of servings you eat from each group.

• You needn't be rigid about it; skipping the meat group on Tuesday or the milk group on Wednesday won't kill you. It's your overall eating patterns that count.

• Fill your plate from the bottom of the pyramid up—starting with plenty of grains, fruits, and vegetables. To get a sense of how your meals should look, divide your plate into four sections. Fill three sections with grains, fruits, and vegetables, and the fourth with a low-fat meat or other protein.

Do Starches Make You Fat?

Health benefits are all well and good, but what lots of people want to know is: Do breads and other grains lead to weight gain? The simple answer: No. In fact, a diet rich in whole grains is apt to do just the opposite. However, there are a couple of easy ways to gain weight on a starchy diet:

• By slathering fats on your bread, baked potato, or pasta;

• By eating too many refined starches such as white bread and cakes, cookies, and pastries.

Instead, go for high-fiber carbohydrates that will fill you up, not out. At least half your grain servings each day should be whole grain. That's three servings a day—minimum. To meet that quota:

• Switch from white bread to whole wheat, particularly seven- or nine-grain whole wheat;

• Buy whole-grain breakfast cereal;

• Opt for whole-wheat pastas over those made with white flour.

The Pyramid's Smart Foods

The Food Guide Pyramid is just an outline of what you should eat; it's up to you to fill in the details. That's both good and not-so-good news: good because it means you can choose from a whole world of foods instead of settling for some rigid regimen, and not-so-good because it means you need to *think* about what you're going to eat.

Every time you walk into the grocery store or

F.Y.I.

To avoid discomfort when you increase your fiber intake, increase it *gradually*, to 20 to 35 grams a day, and drink at least eight cups of water daily.

sit down at a restaurant, you have to decide what you should, and want to, feed your body. Once you familiarize yourself with the smart choices in each food group, however, opting for healthy foods will become second nature.

Bread, Cereal, Rice, and Pasta

This group sits at the bottom of the food pyramid for a reason: Complex carbohydrates are the foundation of a healthy diet.

The stars of this category are whole grains. Most famous for their fiber content, they also contain a range of substances that researchers believe are important to health—substances that are removed from refined grains during processing. Whole grains are rich in vitamin E and other antioxidants—some of which are unique to grains—that may help fend off heart disease and cancer. They also contain compounds that help lower the risk of breast cancer and colon cancer, and researchers believe that a diet rich in whole grains may help prevent adult-onset diabetes.

Best Bets: Bread Group

Whole-Grain Bread
Calories: on average, about 90 per slice; vary with product

Compare bread made with 100 percent whole wheat to plain white bread: The former has three times as much fiber, magnesium, vitamin B6, vitamin E, and chromium, as well as much more zinc, manganese, copper, folic acid, and pantothenic acid (a B vitamin). Not only that, but it tastes better, too.

Be sure to check ingredient labels; don't judge by appearance or even by the words "whole grain," "multigrain," or "made with whole wheat." If the first ingredient on the list is wheat flour or unbleached wheat flour, the bread is mainly refined flour; if the first ingredient is whole-wheat flour (or another whole grain), the bread is primarily whole grain. And look for breads with at least 1.5 grams of fiber per serving.

Oatmeal

Calories: 150 per one cup cooked oatmeal

Fiber-rich oatmeal is helpful in lowering blood cholesterol and the risk of heart disease; it also supplies iron, copper, folic acid, vitamin E, and zinc. And a breakfast bowl of oatmeal will go a long way toward keeping carbohydrate cravings at bay. Oatmeal cookies aren't so bad, either, as cookies go.

Other cereals are a good bet, too: Look for hot cereals with at least 1.5 grams of fiber per serving and ready-to-eat cereals with at least 2.5 grams per serving. Lots of ready-to-eat cereals supply plentiful amounts of zinc and other nutrients. Bran cereals often contain wheat bran or oat bran, which, technically speaking, is not whole grain. But they're still a good source of whole-grain components.

Adding More Grains to Your Life

Here are some tips for enhancing your grain intake:

• Try raisin bran instead of cornflakes.

• Sprinkle some wheat germ, low-fat granola, or low-fat muesli on frozen yogurt or regular yogurt.

• Have a low-fat granola bar as a snack.

• On weekends, make hot oatmeal with a sprinkle of brown sugar.

• Make whole-wheat couscous or quinoa instead of white rice.

• Air-pop popcorn and toss it with Cajun spice mix.

• Instead of a lettuce salad, make a grain salad with bulgur, brown rice, or whole-wheat couscous, tossed with parsley, cucumber, tomatoes, olive oil, salt, and lemon juice.

Carbo Snacks

Choose low-fat or nonfat snacks such as:

Pretzels

Graham crackers

Ginger snaps

Baked tortilla or pita chips

Bagels (but watch out for the gigantic ones—they're pretty calorie-dense)

Brown Rice and Wild Rice

Calories: 216 per one cup cooked brown rice; 248 per one cup cooked wild rice

It's not quite kosher to lump these two together, since wild rice isn't really a rice—it's a seed. But technicalities aside, these two are both wonderful sources of fiber and other nutrients. Brown rice is rich in magnesium, selenium, and antioxidants; the availability of quick-cooking versions leaves you no excuse to stick with white rice. (Even "enriched" white rice is a nutritional weakling.) And wild rice, while pricier and slow-cooking, provides twice as much protein as true rice, along with more riboflavin, niacin, zinc, and other minerals. And its nutty flavor elevates any dish.

Wheat Germ

Calories: 54 per two tablespoons

A fine source of protein, ¼ cup of wheat germ also provides 90 percent of your daily requirements for vitamin E, along with B vitamins, zinc, selenium, manganese, and iron. Sprinkle it on hot cereal or salads or just about any dish to up the nutritional value and add a delicate, nutty flavor; or add it to muffin, bread, or meat loaf batter.

Fruit and Vegetable Groups

The more fruits and vegetables you eat, the better. Not only will you load up on vitamins and minerals and fiber, but you'll fill up on low-fat, low-calorie foods rather than the other kind. It's all well and good to espouse "everything in moderation," but there are times when you crave more—a big, heaping bowl or plateful of something. On top of their many other attributes, fruits and vegetables have something going for them that no other food group can claim: You can pretty much

The Grain Adventure

No need to stick with brown rice night after night: There's a whole exotic world of grains out there to discover. Once a week, try one of the following:

Amaranth: High in protein, calcium, phosphorus, iron, and fiber, as well as amino acids (which are often absent from grain), it has an earthy flavor and a cornmeal-like texture. Eat cooked amaranth as a hot cereal or combine it with other grains and vegetables.

Buckwheat: An earthy-flavored seed that contains high-quality protein, B vitamins, vitamin E, calcium, and iron. Hulled and toasted, it becomes kasha and is great in pilafs and stuffings or combined with vegetables or pasta.

Kamut: Buttery and chewy when cooked, these kernels contain 40 percent more protein than wheat and may be less allergenic. Kamut flour may be substituted for wheat flour in most recipes. Use the cooked whole grain in salads and pilafs.

Millet: A small, nutty-tasting grain that contains high-quality protein as well as potassium, phosphorus, magnesium, and B vitamins. Use in salads and pilafs.

Quinoa: Light and delicate, this seed contains 50 percent more protein and higher levels of iron, phosphorus, and B vitamins than other grains. Use in salads, soups, and pilafs.

Spelt: A nutty, ricelike relative of wheat that's easier to digest and better tolerated by people with wheat allergies. It's got more protein, amino acids, minerals, and B vitamins, too. Substitute spelt flour for whole-wheat flour in baked goods. Use cooked spelt kernels in salads, soups, stews, and veggie burgers.

eat as much as you want! When you are trying to healthy-up and thin down—worrying about portions and fat content and the rest—this news comes as a considerable relief.

Not only *can* you eat lots of fruits and vegetables, you *must*, if you want to be healthy as well as trim. Even when you're cutting calories, you should never skimp on these two food groups. You've probably seen the National Cancer Society's "Eat Five a Day" posters and signs and stickers in your supermarket's produce section. The big push reflects the fact that vitamin- and fiber-rich fruits and vegetables can help reduce the risk of some cancers, heart disease, and other ailments as well as birth defects. There's simply no better source for nutrients.

Some general rules to remember:

• Look for produce that's rich in vitamins A and C, which can help reduce the risk of some cancers and heart disease.

• Choose fruits and vegetables in a wide range of colors to get maximum nutrients.

• Don't get all your fruit servings in juice form; whole fruit gives you fiber as well as vitamins.

Best Bets: Fruit

Note: Fresh fruit is one of the most wonderful things you can eat, both taste- and nutrition-wise. But when it's not handy, opt for dried, frozen, or canned—as long as it's not packed in sweetened syrup.

Citrus Fruit
Calories: 62 per medium orange; 37 per medium tangerine; 37 per half grapefruit

Oranges, tangerines, grapefruit, lemons, and limes: They're all unrivaled sources of vitamin C, fiber, and potassium. Not only that, but the pectin found in citrus fruits may help reduce the risk of heart disease.

Orange juice is a powerhouse in its own right: Although it lacks the dietary fiber of whole fruit, OJ is a quick source of energy that offers not just vitamin C but also a big dose of folic acid, the essential B vitamin that prevents birth defects and possibly cervical cancer. For even more benefits, be sure to buy calcium-fortified juice. And avoid "juice drinks" made with less than 100 percent fruit juice; they're packed with added sugar.

Strawberries
Calories: 45 per cup

A great source of vitamin C, folic acid, B vitamins, potassium, iron, and fiber, strawberries also contain a phytochemical that fights cancer-causing substances. Moreover, they're high in pectin, which reduces cholesterol levels and the risk of hypertension. And what tastes better than a ripe strawberry?

Cantaloupe
Calories: 30 per cup

A cup of cantaloupe provides 125 percent of the daily vitamin C requirement and more than 50 percent for vitamin A; melons may also protect against cancers of the colon and rectum.

Folic Acid

Crucial for preventing birth defects, folic acid is essential during pregnancy. Here are folic acid–rich foods:

Asparagus

Broccoli

Brussels sprouts

Cantaloupe

Spinach

Orange juice

Strawberries

Leafy green vegetables

Fortified breakfast cereals

Raising Your Fruit Profile

Some tips for incorporating more fruits into your life:

• Keep dried fruit, not candy, in your desk drawer or car for easy snacking. But don't overdo it—dried fruits provide concentrated calories along with nutrients.

• Add fruit to your breakfast cereal or on top of yogurt.

• Drink 100 percent fruit juice instead of soda; try a fifty-fifty mix of orange juice and seltzer water to dilute the calories.

• Opt for a fruity dessert rather than a chocolaty one (unless you know you won't be satisfied with anything less than chocolate).

• Drink a glass of juice or eat a piece of fruit first thing in the morning.

• Take a piece of fruit to work each day; then increase to two.

• Be adventurous: Try exotic fruits such as papaya and kiwi, alone or mixed with other fruits in a shake.

Figs
Calories: 200 per 7 dried figs

An excellent source of nutrients, including vitamin B6, potassium, beta-carotene, calcium, magnesium, iron, and fiber, figs are a delicious, satisfying energy source. Some even swear they're an aphrodisiac!

Other good bets:

Apricots, nectarines, and peaches

Berries of all kinds

Watermelon

Mangoes

Papayas

Bananas

Grapes and raisins

Best Bets: Vegetables

The vegetables below are top choices for meeting your daily requirements.

Note: Although frozen vegetables can't compete with fresh when it comes to taste, they are great in terms of convenience and nutrition; in fact, some frozen vegetables contain more of certain nutrients than their fresh counterparts.

Bok Choy
Calories: 24 per cup of cooked bok choy

If you've never even heard of this vegetable, let alone tried it, it's past time to remedy that situation. A member of the cabbage family, bok choy has a mild, crisp flavor and is a great addition to stir-fries. It's a wonderful source of fiber and vitamin A, and a good source of calcium.

Broccoli and Broccoli Rabe
Calories: 44 per cup of steamed broccoli

Broccoli is packed with fiber and folic acid, and a cup's worth gives you almost double your daily vitamin C requirement, as well as vitamins A, B2, and B6, and cancer-fighting phytochemicals. It keeps bones healthy with calcium, potassium, magnesium, and phosphorus. Use frozen broccoli in place of fresh from time to time—it's got more calcium.

Kale
Calories: 42 per cup of cooked kale

A good alternative to the usual spinach, this dark, leafy green is an excellent source of fiber, zinc, and vitamins A, C, and K. Plus it's a better source of absorbable calcium than milk! (As with broccoli, the frozen variety is richer in calcium.)

Sweet Potatoes
Calories: 118 per medium potato

Rich in vitamins C and E, beta-carotene, fiber, potassium, and iron, sweet potatoes also contain cancer-fighting phytochemicals. They're also one of the most satisfying, filling foods you can eat. Don't confuse them with yams, which look similar but lack many of the sweet potato's nutrients.

Upping Your Vegetable Quotient

Ideas for adding more vegetables to your diet:

• Include a salad in one meal a day; not only will it give you extra nutrients, but it will help curb your appetite.

• Buy precut vegetables to toss together into a quick salad.

• Keep vegetables in the front of your refrigerator so you'll reach for them at snack time.

• Be adventurous: Try exotic vegetables such as bok choy or jicama (both great for stir-fries).

• Keep frozen vegetables on hand for convenience; some are more nutritious than fresh vegetables.

• On the run, drink V8 or a similar vegetable juice.

• Grate a carrot into spaghetti sauce to add sweetness and vitamins.

• Skip the pepperoni and order veggie pizza.

Tomatoes

Calories: 26 per medium tomato

For very few calories, tomatoes offer a plenitude of nutritional benefits—not to mention delicious flavor. They're the top source of the antioxidant lycopene, which may help fight cancer; one tomato also packs more than 10 percent of your daily requirement for vitamins A and C, folic acid, and potassium.

Other great choices:

Carrots

Collard greens

Garlic

Onions

Edible seaweed

Spinach

Swiss chard

Watercress

Eat in moderation:

Avocados—they're high in nutrients but also high in fat, albeit the good, monounsaturated kind.

Dairy Group

Foods in the dairy group provide two ingredients that are necessary to a strong, healthy body: protein and calcium, the mineral that's so important for maintaining your bones as well as for regulating your heartbeat, your blood pressure, and nerve impulses.

Unlike fruits and vegetables, however, dairy foods should be eaten in moderation, since they often feature fat along with all that good calcium and protein. Look for low-fat or nonfat versions.

Best Bets: Diary Group

Skim Milk
Calories: 90 per cup

Milk is loaded with calcium, protein, potassium, and riboflavin, and skim milk offers the same nutritional benefits as whole, without the fat. Mixing low-fat or skim milk with nonfat dry milk ups the calcium quotient still further, without adding

SMART DEFINITION

Cruciferous Vegetables
Vegetables in the cabbage family, which contain compounds that can help decrease the risk of some forms of cancer.

The "A" List

The following foods are good to excellent sources of vitamin A, vitamin C, and/or fiber; those marked with an asterisk are also cruciferous. The National Cancer Institute recommends at least one serving of a vitamin A–rich fruit or vegetable and a vitamin C–rich fruit or vegetable daily; at least one serving of a high-fiber fruit or vegetable a day; and several servings of cruciferous vegetables a week.

Apples—fiber
Apricots—A
Asparagus—C
Bananas—fiber
Blackberries—fiber
Blueberries—fiber
Bok choy—A, C*
Broccoli—A, C*
Brussels sprouts—C, fiber *
Cabbage—C*
Cantaloupe—A, C
Carrots—A, fiber
Cauliflower—C*
Cherries—fiber

Collard greens—A*
Dates—fiber
Figs—fiber
Grapefruit—C, fiber
Honeydew—C
Kale—A, C*
Kiwi fruit—C, fiber
Lettuce (romaine, red and green leaf)—A
Mangoes—A, C
Mustard greens—A, C*
Oranges—C, fiber
Papaya—A, C
Pears—fiber
Peppers—C

Pineapple—C
Plums—C
Potatoes—C
Prunes—fiber
Pumpkin—A
Raspberries—fiber
Spinach—A, C, fiber
Squash—A
Strawberries—C, fiber
Sweet potatoes—A, C, fiber
Tomatoes—A, C
Turnip greens—A, C*
Watermelon—C

any fat. And you can add calcium to baked goods, hot cereals, and sauces with evaporated skim milk.

A note about soy milk: If you're lactose intolerant or vegetarian, be sure to drink soy milk that's fortified with calcium; you'd have to drink nearly sixty servings of regular soy milk to get the calcium provided in just one glass of milk.

Low-Fat or Nonfat Yogurt
Calories: 100 per cup of plain nonfat yogurt

As with milk, cutting fat does no damage to the nutritional content of yogurt: In fact, low-fat or nonfat yogurt is a more concentrated source of calcium than whole-milk yogurt, and it offers a good dose of magnesium, potassium, selenium, and vitamins B2 and B12, as well as plenty of protein for relatively few calories—especially if you avoid the more sugar-laden fruit varieties. Active yogurt cultures make it a problem-free food for people with lactose intolerance. And plain, nonfat yogurt makes a great substitute for sour cream, which offers tons of fat and little nutrition.

What about frozen yogurt? It's got a good amount of calcium, too, but it can be loaded with sugar and fat. Opt for low-fat or nonfat frozen yogurt, which has just as much flavor and even more calcium than the full-fat variety.

Hard Cheese

Calories: 114 per ounce of cheddar; 129 per ounce of Parmesan; less for reduced-fat versions

The good news: There's no need to abandon cheese when trying to lose weight. Hard cheeses such as cheddar and Parmesan are a good source of protein and calcium, and the low-fat versions have even more, along with other bone-maintaining minerals. Just don't *eat* them with abandon; watch portions, fat, and sodium content. If you don't like low-fat cheese on its own, mix it half and half with regular cheese.

A Bigger Dose of Dairy

Here are some ideas for adding more dairy to your daily diet:

• Mix nonfat dry milk with skim milk to boost its calcium content and flavor without adding fat.

• Use plain, low-fat or nonfat yogurt on baked potatoes.

• Add evaporated skim milk to cream soups to increase the calcium and flavor quotient.

• Sprinkle low-fat cheese on salads and soups.

• Try adding low-fat or skim milk to your coffee or tea instead of cream or half-and-half. (But if you can't face the day without half-and-half in your coffee, don't beat yourself up about it; just keep it to a minimum and make sure your other dairy choices are low-fat.)

• Make a point of having cereal and milk for breakfast at least three times a week.

The Calcium Connection

Calcium isn't found only in milk products. The antacid Tums provides a whopping 1,250 milligrams of calcium carbonate (500 milligrams of which can be absorbed). Here's a list of best calcium bets, including others that probably will surprise you:

Milk, including lactose-reduced buttermilk

Yogurt

Hard cheese

Cottage cheese

Frozen milk products

Pudding

Mineral water (check labels for calcium-rich brands)

Breads fortified with calcium

Cereals fortified with calcium

Bok choy

Broccoli

Collard greens

Kale

Mustard greens

Okra

Orange juice fortified with calcium

Spinach

Turnip greens

Dried beans

Salmon, canned with bones

Sardines, canned with bones

Tofu prepared with calcium

Low-fat cottage cheese is a good source of protein, but don't look to it for your daily calcium dose: You'd have to eat more than a pint to get the calcium equivalent of one glass of milk.

Ice Cream
Calories: wide variation; look for the nonfat or low-fat versions

Ice cream? On a list of nutritious foods? Well, yes. Ice cream is a very good source of calcium. And while it also packs a punch in terms of fat and calories, you can opt for one of the lower-fat versions; just try to resist the "premium" brands, which have way more fat than the plain old (cheaper) brands. Ice cream is never going to be the best dessert choice, but you could do much worse—especially when you consider the pleasure-per-spoonful quotient. One helpful hint: If you know you can't control yourself around a pintful, go out for a cone when the craving hits, or buy the small individual portion.

Protein Group

Protein foods supply your body with substances needed to build and repair muscles and other tissues. Animal sources provide iron, which helps carry oxygen to muscles, and zinc, which can strengthen your immune system; vegetable proteins offer the added benefits of vitamins, minerals, and fiber.

Most Americans already get more than enough protein in their diet—it's the one food group people don't skimp on—and often the least healthy kinds of protein. The challenge is choosing protein sources that are high in protein but low in unhealthy fats: beans, fish, poultry, and lean meats rather than marbled steaks and fatty lunch meats.

Best Bets: Animal Proteins

Lean Beef
Calories: 230 per 3 ounces lean ground beef; 178 per 3 ounces cooked bottom round

An excellent source of protein, B vitamins, iron,

and zinc, beef can be a dietary boon as long as you are careful to buy only the leanest cuts. (To identify lean cuts, look for those labeled "loin" or "round." Meats labeled "select" are usually the leanest.) Be aware, though, that even lean cuts provide a significant amount of saturated fat and cholesterol; watch your serving sizes.

Chicken

Calories: 142 per 3 ounces cooked white meat; 163 per 3 ounces cooked dark meat

With less fat than most cuts of red meat, chicken is a great choice for health-conscious meat eaters, offering plentiful protein, B vitamins, iron, and zinc. A couple of things to keep in mind:

• White meat is leaner than dark.

• Unless you are cooking a whole chicken, always remove the skin first—it's a major source of fat and cholesterol.

Eggs

Calories: 75 per large egg

No doubt you've heard that eggs are bad news, cholesterol-wise, and maybe you've been steering clear of them for that reason. If so, you're missing out on a terrific source of both protein and lecithin, which is essential to memory, concentration, and emotional balance. Eggs are also rich in zinc and vitamins A, B12, D, and E.

It's true that egg yolks contain a high concentration of cholesterol. But unless you have high levels of blood cholesterol to begin with, dietary cholesterol from foods such as eggs and shellfish is not a threat. (For more on the difference between dietary cholesterol and blood cholesterol, see chapter 3.)

Pacific Salmon

Calories: 175 per 3 ounces cooked salmon; 114 per 3 ounces canned pink salmon

Pacific salmon is not only delicious but also packed with good-for-you fish oil that lowers cholesterol and triglycerides and may raise your levels of "good" (HDL) cholesterol. And canned salmon with bones is an excellent source of calcium. *Note: It's best to stick with Pacific salmon when possible; Atlantic salmon is more likely to be contaminated.*

Although salmon's especially nutrient-rich, you really can't go wrong with any kind of seafood. Other good bets include:

Lobster

Oysters

Sardines

Shrimp

Canned water-packed tuna

Best Bets:
Vegetable Proteins

Unlike animal proteins, vegetable proteins are incomplete—they don't contain all nine essential

Portion Control

When you're trying to eat healthy, keep an eye on fat, and—especially—lose weight, it's essential to know *how much* you are eating. Sounds elementary, but it's very easy to underestimate and end up consuming twice as many servings, as well as twice as much fat and calories, as you intended.

Knowing what "one serving" looks like is tricky when it comes to meat. The Food Guide Pyramid recommends two to three servings of protein a day; here are some examples of what constitutes a serving:

• Half a breast, or leg and thigh, of 2½- to 3-pound chicken.

• Two slices of roast beef or pot roast, 3 × 3 × ¼-inch thick.

• One medium loin pork chop, ¾-inch thick.

• One hamburger patty three inches across and ½-inch thick.

Iron Rich!

Meat products are a particularly excellent source or iron. For good health, select lean meats and skinless poultry most often—they have less fat as well as less saturated fat.

Beef

Veal

Pork

Lamb

Poultry

Clams

Oysters

The iron in plant foods is less available to the body than iron from meat products. To improve iron absorption from plant sources, eat iron foods with a vitamin C–rich food.

Dried beans and peas

Cereals fortified with iron

Breads fortified with iron

Dried figs and raisins

Prune juice

Spinach

amino acids. But that's no cause for concern. By eating a variety of beans, seeds, grains, nuts, and vegetables, you can easily get a variety of complementary proteins, which combine to form complete proteins in your body. It's not necessary to eat complementary proteins at the same meal, but simple combinations such as grains and beans or grains and nuts make it easy to do so.

Dried Beans

Calories: 115 per ½ cup cooked lentils; 125 per ½ cup cooked black beans; 143 per ½ cup cooked garbanzo beans

Dried beans, peas, and lentils are an excellent source of iron and also contain protein and folic acid; high in complex carbohydrates and fiber, they may help lower cholesterol and the risk of cancer. Combined with rice or other starches, they are a mainstay protein source for vegetarians.

Nuts and Seeds

Calories: almonds, 169 per ounce (about a handful); Brazil nuts, 230 per ¼ cup; pecans, 190 per ¼ cup; pumpkin seeds, 72 per ¼ cup; sesame seeds, 223 calories

Calorie for calorie, almonds, Brazil nuts, pecans, pumpkin seeds, and sesame seeds are your best nutritional bets in this category. Although they are high in fat, it's mostly the good kind: monounsaturated or polyunsaturated. You should eat them in moderation, sprinkled on salads, added to poultry dishes or vegetarian meals, or as dessert with a piece of fruit. Here's what they have to offer:

• Almonds: a good protein source, high in vitamin E, some B vitamins, magnesium, and calcium; less fat than other nuts

• Brazil nuts: excellent source of zinc, selenium, and vitamin E

• Pecans: zinc and protein

• Pumpkin seeds: more zinc than any other seed (and zinc-enhancing amino acids, too), plus vitamin E

• Sesame seeds: a good source of calcium—but be sure to chew them well so the minerals are released into your body

Peanut butter is a good protein source, but it takes 6 tablespoons (almost 600 calories!) to get the equivalent of one meat serving. If you're trying to lose weight, you're better off using peanut butter as a condiment—spread on low-fat crackers or celery, for example—than as a protein mainstay. And try the reduced-fat versions.

Tofu
Calories: 88 per 3 ounces

Tofu has more than three times as much iron, magnesium, manganese, and folic acid as red meat, and is a great source of the B vitamins and protein typically supplied by meat—for about half the fat and

Protein's Worst Bets

Bacon

Fast-food hamburgers

Fried fish or chicken

Marbled steaks

Processed meats (such as bologna, salami, sausage)

Bean Bonanza

If you're looking for new culinary frontiers to explore, consider dried beans, which offer amazing variety along with excellent nutritional value. Beans mix well with almost any starch or vegetable and add substance to salads, soups, and casseroles. For convenience at home, buy canned or frozen versions.

• **Adzuki.** Small burgundy beans with a white stripe, with a delicate, sweet flavor and soft texture. Use in soups, salads, stir-fries, and pasta dishes, seasoned with tamari or ginger.

• **Anasazi.** Red and white speckled beans, similar to pinto beans in size, with a sweet, full flavor and mealy texture. Use in Mexican dishes such as refried beans, burritos, and bean dips, seasoned with garlic, cumin, or chiles.

• **Black (turtle).** Small purple-black beans with a mealy texture and earthy taste. Use in sauces, soups, refried beans, salads, and bean dips, seasoned with garlic, lime juice, chiles, cumin, or cilantro.

• **Chickpea (garbanzo).** Medium-size round tan beans with a nutty flavor and firm texture. Use in hummus, soups, and salads, seasoned with olive oil, garlic, lemon juice, parsley, or rosemary.

• **Lentil.** Small yellow, red, green, or brown seeds with an earthy flavor and soft texture. Use in soups, salads, vegetable burgers, and curries, seasoned with onion, garlic, thyme, or curry.

• **Mexican red.** Dark red, similar to a kidney bean but smaller, with a sweet flavor. Use in soups, salads, and chili, seasoned with garlic, onion, chile, and cumin. Substitute for kidney or pinto beans in any recipe.

• **Mung.** Small dark beans with a sweet flavor and soft texture. Use sprouted mung beans in Asian dishes; use regular mung beans in curries, seasoned with tamari, curry, or ginger.

• **White (canellini, great northern, navy).** Cream-colored beans that come in various sizes and have a mild flavor and slightly grainy texture. Use in soups, stews, casseroles, salads, and pasta dishes, seasoned with rosemary and oregano.

calories. It's also a good source of vitamin A and calcium; be sure to buy the firm variety, which is much higher in calcium than the soft kind. Nearly half its calories come from fat, but it's unsaturated fat. You can now find reduced-fat versions as well.

Fats, Oils, and Sugars

The top of the food pyramid is not a place of honor; it's more like Siberia. This is the home of fats, oils, and sugars, foods that offer very little nutritional value and lots of trouble for the weight- and health-conscious.

Fats, oils, and sugars aren't among the five food groups; the USDA offers no recommended number of servings and advises simply: "Eat sparingly." The way to do that is twofold:

• Add less fat and sugar to your foods.

• Avoid "hidden" fats and sugars by opting for natural, unprocessed foods whenever possible.

How Much Fat?

As discussed in chapter 3, your total peak fat "allowance" should be about 30 percent of your daily calories. If you are consuming 1,500 calories, that's 50 fat grams, which equals:

Enhancing Your Protein Quotient

• Add cooked beans to your next salad.

• Put peanut butter on celery (or crackers).

• Add tofu to stir-fried vegetables.

• Snack on nutty trail mix instead of chips.

• Keep sliced turkey and other low-fat deli meats in the refrigerator at home and work.

• Buy tuna or sardines canned in water instead of oil.

• Add strips of grilled lean meat or sliced, skinless poultry to salads.

SMART SOURCES

The growing popularity of wholesome, natural foods should come as no surprise: The health benefits just can't be beat! Here's a source to try as you learn more about foods and nutrition:

The Whole Food Bible: How to Select and Prepare Safe, Healthful Foods Christopher Kilham

• 2 teaspoons oil, mayonnaise, margarine, or butter

• 2 tablespoons diet mayonnaise or margarine

• 2 tablespoons regular salad dressing or 4 tablespoons reduced-fat salad dressing

Cutting the Fat

These guidelines can help you cut the fat and make sure the fat you do eat is the healthiest kind:

• When you do eat fat, try to avoid saturated fat and opt for healthier mono- or polyunsaturated fats, which help lower blood cholesterol. (For more on the difference between them, see chapter 3.) Monounsaturated fats are found in both plant and animal sources; polyunsaturated fats are found mainly in vegetables. Check nutrition labels to find out what you're getting. Canola, olive, and safflower oil are all good choices.

• Butter or margarine? Both are rich sources of saturated fat; neither is going to do your health any good. But if you love butter and can't face your morning toast without it, go ahead and use it—just be careful to use only enough to add flavor. Don't bother switching to margarine; its taste is less satisfying and it contains trans fats, a form of hydrogenated fat that may be especially harmful to your health.

• Switch to reduced-fat or fat-free salad dressings, or use olive oil–based vinaigrette.

• Remember to ferret out hidden fats by reading labels and doing the math. Any food that gets more than a third of its calories from fat should be eaten sparingly. An occasional treat won't do you much damage, but making a habit of it will.

By eating less fat—oil, butter, margarine, salad dressings, cookies, cakes, animal and dairy products—and salty snacks such as chips and nuts, and by eating more fruits, vegetables, and whole-grain breads and cereals, you will lower your risk for cancer, heart disease, diabetes, and many other diseases.

Making Trade-Offs

It's unrealistic to swear off all fatty foods and sweet desserts—and many people would consider life considerably diminished without them. The secret is not abstinence but balance.

You do need to moderate your intake of fat, sugars, and calories in order to get in, and stay in, peak shape. But you can, and should, allow for the occasional indulgence—without an ounce of guilt to go with it.

How? Remember, the Food Guide Pyramid is built on the premise of flexibility. When you choose a food that is higher in fat or sugar, you just need to balance it by making sure your other selections that day (or over the next few days) are better, more-nutritious choices. Although in some ways it's easier to think of a diet that consists of good and bad foods, that attitude won't serve you well in the long run. Moderation and balance add up to a way of eating that lasts a lifetime.

A Word about Chocolate

Consider chocolate. It contains a surprising number of nutrients, including protein, iron, and magnesium, and it is believed to trigger the release of endorphins—"feel good" chemicals—in the brain. It also tastes better than almost anything. And for probably two out of three of these reasons, it's the number one food craved by women.

But there's no question that it belongs at the top of the food pyramid, thanks to its high fat and sugar content. Does this mean you must forever resist it in order to achieve good health? Of course not. When you know it's the only thing that will satisfy your craving, go ahead and indulge. Just do it in moderation, and be sure to cut back on other fatty foods to compensate.

There are smart and less-smart ways to give in to a craving. Where chocolate is concerned, try these minimalist approaches:

• Dip fresh strawberries in low-fat chocolate syrup.

• Have a cup of low-fat, sugar-free hot chocolate.

• Try bittersweet chocolate, which has a wonderfully intense flavor and less sugar.

• Instead of snacking on chocolate, eat it immediately after a meal; you're apt to eat less.

THE BOTTOM LINE

The USDA Food Guide Pyramid encourages you to think in terms of abundant variety, not deprivation, and in terms of nutrition, not just calorie counts. By eating the recommended daily servings, and choosing a range of foods both within and across the six food groups, you'll be sure to get an adequate dose of nutrients and develop a healthy approach to eating.

....

Eating Smart Every Day

Once you have some nutritional knowledge under your belt, it's easy to establish a healthy eating plan. That's not to say it won't require effort: You need to learn new ways of shopping, cooking, and choosing daily menus to meet your health and weight-loss goals, and practice those new habits day in and day out. Soon enough, though, you'll automatically reach for the brown rice instead of the white, choose fruit instead of chips, and sauté food in a teaspoon of olive oil rather than fry it in a vat of fat.

Best of all, you'll learn to like it—not just the way these new habits look and feel on you, but the fresh, light taste of your food, eaten in portions that satisfy you rather than sink you. This chapter will help you get started.

Supermarket Savvy

The best way to eat thin and healthy is by choosing most of your foods from the perimeters of your supermarket—the produce aisle, the dairy case, the fresh meats and fish section, and the bread bakery—with a stop in the grains and legumes aisle. But realistically speaking, you'll probably want to keep using some canned and packaged convenience foods as well. After all, they're not called "convenience" foods for nothing—and many of them not only save you time but are healthy additions to your diet.

Many others, however, are not. How to tell the difference? The USDA has made it easy. New mandatory food labels give you the nutritional lowdown on practically every food on your supermarket shelves. You'll even find this information posted next to many fresh fruit and vegetable displays.

Essential Reading

You probably can think of many better ways to spend your time than reading the backs of jars in your supermarket's spaghetti sauce section. But while nutrition labels will never constitute Great Literature, they are filled with crucial information for the health- and weight-conscious. And once you learn how to read them, you can tell at a glance whether what's inside that can or jar or box is really what you want to be putting in your mouth, all things (fat, cholesterol, lack of redeeming nutritional content) considered.

In the past, food labels often didn't provide complete nutrition information—this information was required only when a food contained added nutrients or when nutrition claims appeared on the label. And when information was supplied, it was often hard to find and read. But today food labels are clear, easy to read, and everywhere you look. Some might even argue they're *too* common: Do you really want to know the nutritional breakdown on one of those bite-size Hershey's chocolate bars? (If not, you're in luck: Hershey's couldn't fit it on the inch-long package—but they do provide an 800 number so you can find out over the phone.) There are times when you just don't want to know how much damage you're doing with one illicit snack or another. But if you force yourself to look, you'll definitely think twice before the next "little indulgence."

LOWFAT MILK

Nutrition Facts

Serving Size 8 fl oz (240 ml)
Servings Per Container 8

Amount Per Serving

Calories 100	Calories from fat 20

	% Daily Value*
Total Fat 2.5g	**4%**
Saturated Fat 1.5g	**8%**
Cholesterol 10mg	**3%**
Sodium 130mg	**5%**
Total Carbohydrate 12g	**4%**
Dietary Fiber 0g	**0%**
Sugars 11g	
Protein 8g	

Vitamin A 10%	•	Vitamin C 4%
Calcium 30%	•	Iron 0%
Vitamin D 25%		

*Percent Daily Values are based on a 2,000 calorie diet. Your daily values may be higher or lower depending on your calorie needs:

		Calories	2,000	2,500
Total Fat	Less than		65g	80g
Sat Fat	Less than		20g	25g
Cholesterol	Less than		300mg	300mg
Sodium	Less than		2,400mg	2,400mg
Total Carbohydrate			300g	375g
Dietary Fiber			25g	30g

Ingredients : Lowfat milk, vitamin A palmitate, vitamin D3

Deciphering Labels

Nutrition information usually appears under the heading "Nutrition Facts" and includes the following information:

Serving Size, Servings per Container, Calories per Serving

In the new nutritional labels, serving size much better reflects people's real eating habits; three chips no longer constitute anyone's idea of "one serving." But it's not necessarily equal to a serving size from the Food Guide Pyramid.

Servings per container tells you how much is in the package and helps you figure out what you've eaten if you consume more than one serving at a time. For example, if a pint of yogurt has four servings per container and you just ate half the carton, you'll know you've had two servings. Doubling the Nutrition Facts information gives you the nutritional content.

Calories from Fat per Serving

If you are into number-crunching, you can use this figure to calculate your daily fat intake—which should not go over 30 percent. Here's how: At the end of the day, add up your total calories and calories from fat. Divide calories from fat by calories. The answer gives you the percentage of calories from fat eaten that day. For example, 450 calories from fat divided by 1,800 calories = 0.25 (25 percent), an amount within the recommended level.

To determine a food's percentage of calories from fat, divide the number of calories from fat by the total calories, then multiply the result by 100.

Tip: To maintain a low-fat diet, make sure most of your foods get no more than 25 percent of their calories from fat.

% Daily Value

Based on a 2,000-calorie diet, this tells you what percent of your daily requirement of each nutrient is provided. For example, if a food provides 1 gram of fat per serving, that translates to 2 percent of your Daily Value, based on a 2,000-calorie diet. Although 2,000 calories may be above your calorie limit when you're trying to lose weight, you still can use the % Daily Value to get a general idea of how high or low a food is in the major nutrients.

If a % Daily Value is less than 10, the food is low in that nutrient. Here's what else to look for:

Fat, Cholesterol, and Sodium

• For total fat, cholesterol, and sodium, the lower the % Daily Value, the better. The same holds true for saturated fat. Unlike monounsaturated and polyunsaturated fats, saturated fat gets its own % Daily Value because of its link to high blood cholesterol and cardiovascular disease.

• Avoid going above 100% Daily Value for sodium, cholesterol, or any type of fat in a single day. If the % Daily Value for any of these is greater than 20 percent, that food will use up a sizable portion of your daily quota. That doesn't mean you should avoid it, but you should adjust your eating accordingly.

F.Y.I.

When you compare the nutritional value of two products, make sure the serving sizes are about the same. If not, the comparison won't be valid.

WHAT MATTERS, WHAT DOESN'T

What Matters

• When you're trying to lose weight, the % Daily Values for fat and fiber are most important. If the % Daily Values are 5 or less, the food is considered low in that nutrient. So ideally the foods you choose should have a % Daily Value of 5 or less for fat and 5 or more for fiber.

What Doesn't

• The nutritional claims a product makes on the front of the package—unless they are backed up by the information on the Nutrition Facts label.

• No more than 10 percent of your day's calories should come from saturated fat.

Total Carbohydrates, Fiber, and Sugars

• The % Daily Value for carbohydrates comes from all kinds of carbs, including sugars and dietary fiber. Keep in mind that carbohydrates should make up about 60 percent of your daily calories.

• If the total number of grams of carbohydrates is more than double that of sugars, the food is high in complex carbohydrates, the kind most important to a healthy diet. There's no % Daily Value for sugars; the content is given in grams. (For comparison purposes, keep in mind that a packet of sugar contains 4 grams.)

• A high % Daily Value for fiber is very desirable. If a label indicates 10 percent or more of the % Daily Value for fiber, the food's a good source. Many packaged foods contain no fiber, so if it's even listed on the label, that's something. You should be aiming for 20 to 35 grams a day, so every bit counts.

Protein and Other Nutrients

There's no % Daily Value given for protein; the content is listed in grams. The USDA recommends that women twenty-five or older get about 50 grams a day; men the same age should eat about 63 grams. If the number of protein grams on a label is more than 20 percent of your daily recommendation, the food is a good source of protein.

Vitamin and mineral content is listed as well:

Good sources of nutrients fall between 10 and 19 percent of the Daily Value. If a food provides 20 percent or more of the Daily Value for any vitamin or mineral, it's an excellent source.

Nutritional Claims

On the front of food packages, you'll often find bold face claims such as "fat-free," "low calorie," and "high fiber." Don't judge the food's nutritional merits by such claims; always check the Nutrition Facts label for the whole story. It's the overall nutritional profile that counts. For example, "low-fat" cakes and cookies may still be high in calories because of added sugar. And "high fiber" granola may be loaded with fat.

Fresh Food Tips

As you load your shopping cart with nutritious fruits and vegetables (see chapter 5 for the top choices), keep these pointers in mind:

• Buy only the freshest fruits and vegetables; they should be bright and crisp, without bruising or browning. As often as possible, choose native, seasonal produce—you'll get foods at their best quality and price at the peak of their season. Most fresh vegetables can be stored for two to five days, and root vegetables can be stored from one to several weeks.

Label Lingo

Labels can no longer make claims willy-nilly; terms such as "low-fat" or "reduced-fat" now must reflect uniform standards set by the USDA. Below are translations for the most common packaging claims:

Nonfat: No fat

Fat free: Less than 0.5 gram of fat per serving

Low fat: 3 grams or less per serving, and if the serving size is 30 grams or less or 2 tablespoons or less, per 50 grams of the food

Reduced or less fat: At least 25 percent less per serving than the original food

Low saturated fat: Less than one gram of saturated fat per serving

Low cholesterol: Less than 20 milligrams and less than 2 grams of saturated fat

Low sodium: Less than 140 milligrams of sodium

Very low sodium: Less than 35 milligrams of sodium

Lean (meat, poultry, or fish): Less than 10 grams of fat, 4.5 grams or less of saturated fat, and less than 95 milligrams of cholesterol per serving and per 100 grams

Extra lean: No more than five grams of fat, two grams or less of saturated fat, and no more than 95 milligrams of cholesterol per serving and per 100 grams

Calorie free: Fewer than 5 calories per serving

Low calorie: 40 or fewer calories per serving, or, if the serving is 30 grams or less or 2 tablespoons or less, per 50 grams of the food

Reduced or fewer calories: At least 25 percent fewer calories per serving than the original food

High: Contains at least 20 percent of the Daily Value of whatever nutrient the food is "high" in

Light or "lite": At least one-third fewer calories or half or less the fat of the original food—but only if the original food gets 50 percent or more of its calories from fat; *or* a low-calorie, low-fat food whose sodium content has been reduced by 50 percent or more than the original food

High fiber: 5 grams or more per serving

Good source of fiber: 2.5 grams to 4.9 grams per serving

More or added fiber: At least 2.5 grams more per serving than the original food

Sugar free: Less than 0.5 gram per serving

No added sugar, without added sugar, no sugar added: No sugar or ingredients containing sugars (such as fruit juices, applesauce, or dried fruit) added during processing or packing; no ingredients made with added sugars, such as jams, jellies, or concentrated fruit juice; if the total calories are not reduced, a statement will appear next to the no-sugar claim explaining that the food is "not low-calorie" or "not for weight control"; if calories are reduced, the claim must be accompanied by a "low-calorie" or "reduced-calorie" claim.

Reduced sugar: At least 25 percent less sugar than the original food

Healthy: Low in fat and saturated fat, with only small amounts of cholesterol and sodium; the food must also have at least 10 percent of one or more of the following: vitamin A, vitamin C, iron, calcium, protein, or dietary fiber; if it's a frozen entrée, it must meet at least two of these requirements to qualify as "healthy"

Good source of: Contains at least 10 percent of the Daily Value of that nutrient

Fresh: Unprocessed, never frozen or heated, no preservatives—though it can have undergone irradiation; "fresh frozen," "frozen fresh," and "freshly frozen" mean food that was frozen while still fresh

Irradiated: A food that has been exposed to low doses of radiation to kill organic contaminants and extend its shelf life without affecting color, flavor, or nutrition

• If you shop only once a week, buy a mixture of ripe and unripe fresh produce as well as frozen fruit and vegetables and juices. Eat the fresh items first, starting with the ripest; save the processed foods for later in the week.

• Watch out for supermarket salad bars. They can be a good source of quick-meal ingredients, but don't think that because a food is called "salad" it's necessarily good for you. Choose plain fruits and vegetables, which you can eat as a salad or for snacks, in stir-fry dishes, or in soups. For dressing, choose oil and vinegar or lemon juice. Avoid high-fat items such as potato salad, macaroni salad, and coleslaw.

The following tips will help you make the healthiest choices in the meat, poultry, and fish departments:

• Select meat with the least amount of visible fat— it should have little marbling (fat in the muscle tissue) and not much fat around the edges.

• Look for the words "round" and "loin"; these are lower-fat cuts of meat.

• Buy extra-lean (90 percent lean) ground beef.

• Avoid high-fat processed meats such as bologna, frankfurters, salami, and bacon. Use chicken, turkey, or tuna as sandwich fillings instead.

• With poultry, white meat is leaner than dark.

• For the freshest fish, go to a store that specializes in seafood. Fresh fish should have a firm texture and no "fishy" smell.

A Well-Stocked Pantry

If you keep your kitchen supplied with these healthy staples, along with a variety of fresh foods, you'll always have the makings of a satisfying, nutritious meal or snack.

Bottled Products
Dressings, fat free and
   reduced fat
Extracts: almond,
   vanilla, peppermint
100-percent-fruit spreads
Honey
Dijon mustard
Low-sodium soy sauce
Rice, red wine, and bal-
   samic vinegars

Herbs and Spices
Note: Fresh herbs are best,
but keep the dried version
on hand, too.
Basil
Cayenne pepper
Cinnamon: stick and
   ground
Cloves
Coriander
Cumin
Curry powder
Dill
Dry mustard
Ginger
Oregano
Pepper
Red pepper flakes
Rosemary
Sage

Salt
Sesame seeds
Tarragon
Thyme

Canned and Packaged
Goods
Almonds
Dried apricots
Artichoke hearts
   (packed in water)
Baking powder
Baking soda
Dried or cooked canned
   beans: black, gar-
   banzo, pinto
Multigrain and bran
   cereals
Low-sodium chicken
   broth
Cocoa powder
Ginger snap cookies
Couscous
Fat-free crackers
Whole-wheat flour
Low-fat granola
Hummus
Lentils
Dried mushrooms
Nonstick cooking spray
Oatmeal
Olive oil

Parmesan cheese
Pasta (particularly
   whole wheat)
Reduced-fat peanut
   butter
Pimientos
Popcorn
Prunes
Raisins and currants
Brown and wild rice
Canned salmon
Salsa
Sardines
Low-fat spaghetti sauce
Tabasco
Low-sodium, low-fat
   canned soups
Water-packed tuna
Sparkling water
Tea
Baked tortilla chips

Frozen Foods
Strawberries, raspber-
   ries, and cranberries
Whole-grain waffles
Broccoli, collard greens,
   spinach, and other
   leafy greens (to supplement fresh versions)
Vegetable and chicken
   broth

The Joy of Cooking Thin

Making meals from scratch is a great boon to your weight-loss efforts. For one thing, it's by far the best way to control what goes into your food. It's also a wonderful way to have fun and experiment with meals, allowing you to see that "dieting" does not have to mean a bland, boring regimen; when you prepare recipes from scratch instead of relying on prepared foods, the opportunities for experimenting and adventure are limitless.

If you enjoy cooking, the only challenge is unlearning some unhealthy habits and adding a new repertoire of techniques and ingredients. But if you've never cooked much before, don't worry: Many of the healthiest dishes require little more than throwing together a few fresh ingredients—the simpler, the better. It's completely up to you to decide whether you want to start getting fancy. Once you stop relying on a diet of convenience foods and start experimenting in the kitchen, you may find you enjoy cooking almost as much as eating!

Some Simple Rules

There are three basic requirements for making healthy, calorie-conscious meals:

• Use lots of whole grains, fresh produce, low-fat dairy products, and lean proteins.

• Supplement fresh foods with nutritious processed and packaged foods.

• Cook with minimal added fat.

You'll find a plethora of low-fat, health-conscious cookbooks at your local bookstore, which will give you a much more useful range of recipes than could be squeezed into these pages. Most such recipes rely on fundamental guidelines of healthy cooking, which emphasize low-fat preparation methods and substitutions. Once you know the tricks and techniques, it's easy to turn your old recipes into healthy but great-tasting new ones. For example:

• Instead of frying foods, try cooking them over low to medium-low heat, which reduces the need for added oil and keeps meats and vegetables from overcooking on the outside. You can make "fried" potatoes this way, using cooking spray and a little water in a nonstick pan. You can even make chicken that's as satisfying as fried by soaking skinless chicken pieces in ice water for a couple of hours, rolling them in seasoned bread crumbs, and cooking them over very low heat in a nonstick pan until almost done, then turning up the heat for a few minutes to finish cooking the chicken and to brown the outside.

• To make low-fat meat loaf, add lots of diced vegetables to a pound of ground sirloin, and cook it in a pan with a perforated bottom so that fat can drain out.

• If you're craving lasagna, try using vegetables or black beans instead of meat. Save some fat by switching from regular mozzarella to reduced-fat mozzarella. To save more fat, substitute low-fat cottage or ricotta cheese for whole-milk ricotta.

SMART SOURCES

The following magazines offer clear guidance and abundant ideas for flavorful, low-fat cooking:

Cooking Light Magazine
Southern Living, Inc.
2100 Lakeshore Dr.
Birmingham, AL 35209
800-336-0125

Eating Well: The Magazine of Food and Health
P.O. Box 52919
Boulder, CO 80322-2919
800-678-0541

Flavor Secrets

It is not only possible, but easy, to add flavor with little or no fat. Some ideas:

• Toss carrots with orange juice and a sprinkle of orange zest before baking.

• Top baked potatoes with Dijon mustard instead of butter.

• Mix horseradish and nonfat yogurt into tuna.

• Spread a mixture of low-fat mayonnaise and lemon juice on fish before broiling; serve sprinkled with parsley.

• Sprinkle a teaspoon of grated Parmesan on steamed green beans.

• Steam vegetables with chicken broth.

Such experiments can be a hit-or-miss proposition, however. If you try substituting lower-fat ingredients in prepared cake mixes—such as applesauce for oil, and egg whites for whole eggs—the finished product can fall flat. You may be better off with a mix packaged as "reduced-fat" or "fat-free" because these mixes have been reformulated. Or bake from scratch using a low-fat cookbook. Or buy a single-serving portion of your favorite decadent dessert and enjoy every bite—just cut back on your fat and sugar intake elsewhere to compensate.

Cutting the Fat

Below are some simple ways you can reduce fat and calories in your everyday cooking.

• Reduce the amount of fat in recipes by one-third to one-half, and use polyunsaturated and monounsaturated oils.

• When using recipes that call for more than one egg, substitute two egg whites for each additional whole egg.

• Use skim or low-fat milk to make sauces, puddings, and baked goods.

• Substitute evaporated skim milk in recipes calling for regular evaporated milk.

• Try undiluted evaporated milk instead of cream.

• Use plain low-fat yogurt or whipped cottage cheese as a substitute for sour cream in dips or salad dressings.

• Drain plain low-fat yogurt in a strainer lined with cheesecloth. Season the drained yogurt with herbs and use as a spread in place of cream cheese.

• Substitute plain low-fat yogurt for some of the salad dressings or mayonnaise in recipes.

• Try low-fat cheeses, such as part-skim ricotta or mozzarella. (When cooking, add cheese last so that it does not become tough and stringy during cooking.)

• Trim visible fat from meat. Cutting the fat off a 3-ounce piece of broiled sirloin steak lowers fat from 15 grams to 6 grams and calories from 240 to 150.

• Remove skin from poultry either before (for chicken pieces) or after (for roasted whole chicken) cooking. Taking the skin off a half breast of roasted chicken reduces fat from 8 grams to 3 grams and calories from about 195 to 140.

• Use low-fat marinades to enhance flavor and increase tenderness of meat and poultry. To marinate, let meat stand in a seasoned liquid in the refrigerator for a few hours or overnight. For example, marinate a pound of round steak in a mixture of 2 tablespoons tarragon vinegar and ¼ cup orange juice seasoned with 1 tablespoon Worcestershire sauce, ¼ teaspoon garlic powder, ⅛ teaspoon pepper, and ¼ cup sliced onion.

SMART SOURCES

The following books offer hundreds of healthy, low-fat recipe ideas:

The Wellness Lowfat Cookbook
The Editors of the University of California at Berkeley Wellness Newsletter

Cut the Fat: More Than 500 Easy and Enjoyable Ways to Reduce Fat from Every Meal
The American Dietetic Association

The Pyramid Cookbook: Pleasures of the Food Guide Pyramid
Pat Baird

Jane Brody's Good Food Book: Living the High-Carbohydrate Way
Jane Brody

• Broil, roast, or bake meats instead of frying. To prevent drying and add flavor, baste with wine, lemon or tomato juice, or a low-fat broth rather than fatty drippings.

• Stir-fry thinly sliced meats in a small amount of oil, using a nonstick pan or wok.

• Chill meat juices and skim off fat before adding to stews, soups, and gravies.

• Brown ground meats without added fat. Drain off fat before mixing in other ingredients.

• Place meat on a rack when roasting, broiling, or braising so that fat can drain away from the meat.

• Use commercially prepared sauces, such as barbecue sauce, sparingly. These are often high in sugars, sodium, or both.

Putting It All Together

Now you know the basics: the best foods to eat and how to prepare them. The question: How do you incorporate all this into an easy-to-live-with eating plan?

Here's a simple two-step plan:

1. At first, follow a preplanned menu that ensures you will get a well-balanced variety of foods that does not exceed your daily calorie limit.

2. After a couple of weeks, devise your own free-form eating plan based on the Food Guide Pyramid.

When you're just getting started on a new weight-loss effort, it's important to establish a system to track your eating. Haphazard eating often leads to overeating; planning helps you keep track of what you're consuming and make sure you're getting a nutritious balance of foods. And it helps you learn how much you can eat without going over your daily calorie limit. Pretty soon you will know what a portion looks like and whether you can afford a cup of rice or half a cup of rice with dinner. Starting with a planned daily menu is akin to using training wheels for the first couple of weeks.

But even in the beginning, there's no need to follow menus to the letter. You can substitute similar foods and otherwise adapt the meals to fit your preferences and lifestyle.

The sample menus are based on a daily diet of about 1,500 to 1,600 calories. Because the goal is to make healthy choices, not count every calorie, these menus don't include calorie breakdowns for each food. But if you are determined to know, you can get a good idea by checking the calorie chart at the back of this book.

A diet of 1,500 or 1,600 calories a day will help most mildly to moderately active women lose about a pound or a pound and a half per week. If you find you're not losing at that rate, you can adjust your intake accordingly. You'll find suggestions for adding and subtracting calories following the menus.

Healthy Menus to Get You Started

You can mix and match these breakfast, lunch, and dinner menus as you like. You also can substitute similar foods for those listed—check the Food Guide Pyramid first to make sure you choose another appropriate food from the same group.

Breakfast Menus

1 cup calcium-fortified orange juice
2 whole-grain waffles
½ cup nonfat vanilla yogurt
½ cup blueberries

Fruit cup made with ½ cantaloupe, cut in cubes, and 1 cup orange sections
Small bran muffin
2 teaspoons jam
1 cup skim or 1% milk (in coffee, tea, or alone)

1 cup calcium-fortified orange juice
1 cup cooked oatmeal
1 cup skim or 1% milk (in coffee, tea, or alone)
1 cup berries

½ grapefruit
2 slices whole-grain bread
2 teaspoons jam
1 cup skim or 1% milk (in coffee, tea, or alone)

½ sliced mango
Small bagel with 1 tablespoon low-fat
  cream cheese
1 cup skim or 1% milk (in coffee, tea,
  or alone)

Lunch Menus

*Note: At lunch, dinner, and in between,
mineral water or spring water are your best
beverage options; remember, your goal is to
drink at least eight 8-ounce glasses of water
a day.*

Salad bar: leafy greens (romaine,
  spinach; arugula, mesclun, and
  others); ⅓ cup garbanzo beans;
  shredded carrots and other unmar-
  inated vegetables; 1 hard-boiled
  egg; and 2 tablespoons low-fat or
  fat-free dressing
2 slices whole-grain bread
1 piece fresh fruit

1 cup tomato soup
Turkey sandwich: 2 ounces turkey
  breast, mustard, lettuce, and tomato
  on whole-grain bread
1 piece fresh fruit

1 cup split pea or lentil soup
2 slices whole-grain bread
1 cup fresh fruit salad

Grilled cheese sandwich: 2 ounces reduced-fat
  or low-fat cheddar and 2 tomato slices and one
  red-onion slice in 2 slices of whole-grain

Satisfying Snacks

The best low-calorie snacks are low in fat and sugar and provide fiber and nutrients such as vitamins, minerals, and protein. Try the following:

Low-fat pretzels

Fat-free yogurt or plain yogurt with a teaspoon of honey or fresh fruit

Baked tortilla chips with salsa

Air-popped popcorn

Carrot and celery sticks

Angel food cake

Rice cakes with a tablespoon of all-fruit preserves

Frozen banana slices

Whole-grain cereal

bread rubbed with ½ teaspoon olive oil and grilled in a nonstick skillet

Green salad (as much as you want; try to include romaine and spinach leaves) with 2 tablespoons low-fat or fat-free vinaigrette

1 piece fresh fruit

Baked potato with ½ cup broccoli and 1 ounce shredded reduced-fat cheddar cheese

1 cup fruit salad

Dinner Menus

3 ounces grilled salmon

½ cup steamed broccoli

1 whole-wheat roll

¾ cup low-fat frozen yogurt (no more than 110 calories per half cup)

1 cup cooked whole-wheat pasta with ½ cup tomato sauce (containing no more than 3 grams of fat per ½ cup) and 2 teaspoons Parmesan cheese

Green salad (as much as you want; try to include romaine and spinach leaves) with 2 tablespoons low-fat or fat-free dressing

1 slice whole-wheat garlic bread made with 1 teaspoon olive oil, fresh-pressed garlic, and pepper

4 ginger snap cookies

1 cup vegetarian chili

¾ cup cooked brown rice

Green salad (as much as you want; try to include romaine and spinach leaves) with 2 tablespoons low-fat or fat-free dressing

1 cup fruit salad

½ breast (about 4 ounces) broiled chicken, skin
    removed
1½ cups steamed vegetables
1 medium sweet potato
1 baked apple with cinnamon

Vegetarian stir-fry with 3 ounces cubed tofu and 1
    cup vegetables
¾ cup cooked brown rice
½ mango and ½ papaya, cubed and mixed with
    lemon juice and honey

Healthy Snacks and Add-Ons

Remember, your goal is to lose a healthy one to
one and a half pounds a week. If you find you're
losing too quickly and your energy is flagging, you
should up your daily calories to the next level—
say, 1,700—which should allow you to keep losing
while providing you with more stamina.

If you're losing at a good rate and feeling fine,
except for a constant gnawing hunger in your
stomach, you can add a little extra to your daily
intake—either during or between meals. Adding
complex carbohydrates to your meals can help
give you a "full" feeling: Try an extra slice of
whole-grain bread, ⅓ cup cooked rice, or a cup of
cereal. If you're still hungry, add an extra fruit or
vegetable serving.

Snacks get a bad rap when it comes to weight
loss—in fact, as long as you choose wisely and
keep track of your intake, a snack here and there
can do more to sustain than to sabotage your diet.
On the other hand, how many people do that?
Snacking tends to be a mindless, instant-gratifica-
tion-oriented activity—and as you've figured out

by now, that sort of behavior has no place in your new eating plan. This doesn't mean you can't eat snacks that simply taste good now and then. You can—you just need to plan for them. And make them the exception, not the rule.

Most of your snacks should be a healthy addition to your daily menu, not a detour into the empty-calorie zone. Here are some savvy ideas:

• Banana smoothie: In a blender combine 1 ripe banana, ½ cup skim milk, and ½ cup low-fat vanilla frozen yogurt.

• Hot cocoa made with skim milk and reduced-calorie cocoa mix.

• V8 or other vegetable juice—it'll help fill you up before a meal.

Don't forget: Calories and fat count no matter when or how you eat them, even lying on the couch or standing in front of the refrigerator. So be sure to factor in your snacks when tallying up your daily intake. And by the way, stop eating in front of the refrigerator; whenever possible, sit down when you eat, even if you're eating a snack. Not only can you taste and enjoy your food much better that way, but you'll also be much more aware of how much you're eating.

Turn to chapter 7 for tips on replacing empty-calorie snacks with nutritious alternatives.

Small Meals

Another way to keep your energy up and hunger pangs at bay is by eating four to six small meals a day, rather than the traditional "three squares."

However, don't believe the common wisdom that eating small meals will speed up your metabolism, forcing your body to burn more calories. While researchers have found that animals store less fat when they're fed smaller, more frequent meals, this has never been demonstrated to be the case with humans. And there's no truth to the notion that large meals "overload" your system. True, your body can use only so much food at one time, and extra calories are stored as fat. But your body uses that stored fat when it needs energy; if you're burning all the calories you take in, you won't store fat permanently.

One good argument against frequent meals: Government studies have found that the more times a day people eat, the more calories they tend to consume. So if you're going to try this approach, you need to be particularly vigilant about your intake. For at least the first couple of weeks on your new eating plan, you're best off sticking with the basic three meals a day, as outlined in this chapter. When you begin devising your own menus, based on the Food Guide Pyramid (more on that ahead), you can easily split up your daily intake into four to six meals if you prefer. Some valid reasons to do so:

• Your energy droops late in the day. If so, try having a lighter lunch and another small meal in the mid-afternoon. A mini-meal that combines carbo-

Are You Really Hungry?

Before you grab a snack or clean off every bite on your plate, stop and ask yourself that simple question. Jane Hurley, senior nutritionist at the Center for Science in the Public Interest, says, "We tend to use the food on our plate instead of the way our stomach feels as the standard for how much we should eat." It comes back to paying attention to your body's signals. Being mindful—not only of what you are eating but whether you are eating it for the right reason (because you are hungry)—is one of the most crucial components of successful weight loss.

Anti-Deprivation Desserts

• Squeeze lime or lemon over a fruit salad.

• Alternate layers of fresh fruit with vanilla low-fat yogurt.

• Bake or broil a pear or apple, sprinkled with cinnamon or nutmeg.

• Put an unpeeled ripe banana on a cookie sheet and bake at 350°F for 20 minutes. Split with a knife; sprinkle with cinnamon.

hydrates, fat, and protein—such as fruit and cheese—will give you more sustained energy than a single-food snack.

• Your doctor says your energy lags are due to hypoglycemia. If so, eating more frequently will improve your energy and focus. Frequent small meals also help diabetics regulate blood-sugar levels.

If you decide to go the mini-meal route, be sure to do it the smart, nutritious way. Instead of filling up on empty-calorie snacks, keep healthy ingredients within easy reach at home, at work, and in the car. Try whole-wheat crackers, reduced-fat peanut butter, and raisins. And don't forget to listen to your body. Eat only because you are hungry, not because you ate yesterday at this time.

The Pyramid Plan

When you are ready to start devising your own daily menus, keep the following guidelines in mind:

• Begin by eating the minimum number of suggested servings from each group in the Food Guide Pyramid:

Bread group: 6 servings
Vegetable group: 3 servings
Fruit group: 2 servings
Dairy group: 2 servings
Meat group: 2 servings

This will give you an average daily intake of 1,500 to 1,600 calories—or a little less or more depending on the foods you choose.

• Try not to use more than 2 teaspoons added fat a day; your total daily fat should not exceed 50 grams.

• To keep track of your intake for the first week or so, keep a checklist on which you can mark off the servings you eat from each category. This can get tricky when you're eating something other than a plain piece of fish or a slice of bread. A chicken fajita, for example—what food group does it fit in? When you eat a combination food like this—or pizza, casseroles, pasta salads, and many others—simply break it down into its components. For the fajita, you can figure 1 meat serving (3 ounces of chicken), 1 bread serving (a flour tortilla), ½ dairy serving (3 tablespoons of low-fat cheese), and 1 vegetable (combining the chopped tomato, onion, and lettuce). No, you don't have to keep doing painstaking calculations for the rest of your life, but it's a good idea right now, when you need to learn to pay attention to every bite.

F.Y.I.

Keep in mind that you need a minimum number of calories each day just to stay healthy. No matter how much weight you want to lose or how impatient you are to lose it, don't go below 1,200 calories a day without consulting a physician.

F.Y.I.

Research at Georgia State University and Monell Chemical Senses Center in Philadelphia has shown that people who drink calorie-containing beverages with or between meals consume more calories overall than those who drink water or other noncaloric beverages. So although low-fat milk and juice are great dietary staples, beware of how much you are drinking—they have 80 to 130 calories a cup, which is more than a low-calorie soda. And watch out for sweetened iced tea and seltzers, tonic water, and lemonade, too—unlike milk and juice, they offer mainly empty calories.

Checklist for Healthy Menus

1. Does a day's menu provide at least the lower number of servings from each of the major food groups?

2. Do menus for a week include several servings of dark green leafy vegetables (such as broccoli, kale, spinach, romaine lettuce)? Dry beans or peas (kidney beans, split peas, lentils)?

Remember: Although the pyramid plan gives you almost endless flexibility—you can eat three meals, six meals, or nothing but snacks, if you like—you still need to be careful about sticking to the number of servings and portion sizes on your checklist.

Daily Eating Do's and Don'ts

Here are some more tips for keeping your eating plan on track:

• Don't let yourself feel deprived. If you're used to filling up your plate, keep doing so—just use a smaller plate. A salad plate works very well. Or fill the "blank" spots on your plate with salad greens.

• Do try to eat your meals without distractions—particularly the TV.

• Don't skip breakfast. If you do, you're apt to overcompensate by eating more over the course of the day. Plus, research shows that breakfast eaters have faster reaction times, higher productivity during late-morning hours, and less fatigue. If you can't bear to eat first thing in the morning, wait an hour and then have a piece of fruit, followed half an hour later by toast or some yogurt.

• Do eat slowly. It's better for your digestion, and it allows your body to register that you've eaten something.

• Do try to limit caffeine to two cups of coffee, two glasses of iced tea, or two diet sodas per day.

THE BOTTOM LINE

There's no way around it: Smart, everyday eating requires thought and planning. But once you learn the basics of shopping, cooking, and menu planning, it's easy to make every meal count toward your thin, healthy goals.

Danger Zones

• Learning and adopting smart restaurant strategies will benefit your weight-loss plan and allow you the pleasures of dining out and socializing.

• Navigating holidays, parties, and other choppy waters need not be catastrophic to your efforts.

• There are ways to deal with compulsive snacking without leaving you feel deprived and hungry.

• Controlling alcohol intake is important to your program as well as to your health.

• Being successful means learning to recognize "mood" eating and adjusting your habits to break the destructive patterns.

So you know all about what you *should* eat, and you're savvy about shopping and stocking your kitchen with healthy foods. But what about when you step outside your door—to a restaurant, a ball game, a movie? Or when other people in your household aren't as enamored of fat-free as you are? If you're terrified of losing control in the face of temptation, relax—and read on.

The Pleasures and Perils of Eating Out

Thanks to busy work schedules and activity- and travel-intensive lifestyles, the average American now eats out about 213 times a year, or four times a week, consuming almost 30 percent of his or her calories away from home. What this means, if you're anywhere near the average, is that you can't afford to think of eating out as a "special occasion" during which the rules of healthy eating don't apply. If you let yourself go 213 times a year, your body's going to be in big trouble.

Eating out encompasses a vast range of activities, from sitting down in a fancy restaurant to grabbing a burger at a fast-food joint to eating a hot dog at the neighborhood street fair. All can involve some serious eating dilemmas, unless you keep your dietary wits (those you amassed in previous chapters) about you.

Restaurant Roulette

Many people do their most serious, intensive eating at restaurants, where ordering four times as much as you usually eat somehow seems quite normal—and is certainly encouraged. Consider your average Italian restaurant: It's not unusual to work through bread, appetizers, salad, and a pasta course *before* you even get to the entrée. And then there's the Chianti, the cannoli, and the cappuccino and cookies.

Basically, you've got two options when dining out: Eat what you want, and then balance it out over the next day or two with meals that are lower in calories, fat, sodium, sugars, and alcohol. This works best, of course, if you eat out only occasionally. If you're really going for a big night out, a special-occasion meal, that's one thing. *Mangia!* Enjoy yourself! And plan on eating low-fat as well as exercising tomorrow.

But if you eat out on a regular basis, you can't let your good eating habits fall by the wayside just because you are not eating food you prepared yourself. Instead, you need to choose carefully, trying to maintain your healthy diet as much as possible. That applies not only at sit-down restaurants but at fast-food eateries and anywhere else you may grab a bite. Although you'll have much less control over how foods are prepared and what ingredients are used when you eat out, you still can control which dishes you order and the amount you eat. Just as at home, it's a matter of conscious eating.

SMART MONEY

Jeremy Iggers, author of *The Garden of Eating*, offers this advice: "When you eat mindfully, pausing to take note of the flavor and the texture of the food, and of the sensations on the tongue, you're likely to eat more slowly, and to eat less."

Dining-Out Strategies

Making menu selections *can* be bewildering. Based on the type of restaurant you're visiting, you'll probably have some idea of what to expect, but unless it's a place you visit regularly, you're still likely to face a menu full of unknown quantities. Even the simplest items can vary wildly from one establishment to another in terms of preparation method. And it's easy to be bewildered in ethnic restaurants, where portions, ingredients, and courses may be all over the map, so to speak.

The number-one dictum: Ask—and you shall receive (most of the time).

Don't leave it to chance; ask your waitperson to explain how the food is prepared and find out whether the kitchen will make adjustments or substitutions. For example, you might ask:

• What size are the servings? Can you get a half-order or smaller portion?

• Are meat, chicken, and fish broiled with butter or other fat? Can yours be prepared without added fat?

• Can chicken be prepared without the skin?

• Are the vegetables fresh? How are they prepared?

• Can you get dressings and sauces on the side?

• Can salt or other unwanted ingredients be omitted when your food is prepared?

• Can you get healthier options not listed on the menu?

If you're worried about making a pest of your-self, call the restaurant ahead of time and ask if it will honor special requests. (Do try to keep these reasonable, though; don't go to a barbecue joint and ask them to hold the sauce.)

More Tips for Smart Dining

Keep in mind that it's all a matter of balance. There's really nothing you *can't* order when eating out. If you're desperate for a cheese-smothered enchilada at your favorite Mexican joint, don't bother trying to make do with a small salad. Order the one item you want most, and if it happens to be one that's loaded with fat and calories, split it with a friend or immediately ask the waiter to wrap half of it to go. (Some people opt for dousing their unwanted portion with salt or sugar. Try to save this wasteful tactic for emergencies.) And concentrate on eating low-fat foods the next day.

A wise strategy: Whenever possible, order one course at a time. When you've finished it, if you're still hungry, order another. Granted, this is not always convenient, especially at restaurants that serve more elaborate, time-consuming dishes. But at others it's no problem, and you may ending up eating a *lot* less.

The following are some more helpful tips, arranged course by course.

The Bread Basket

This poses a dilemma. These days, bread baskets are often filled with all sorts of delicious, good-for-you whole-grain breads. Even when you're faced with a basket of plain old white bread, you may be

SMART MONEY

Here's a good strategy to cut fat and increase vegetable intake, from Graham Kerr, former host of television's *Galloping Gourmet* and author of *Minimax Cookbook*: "Whatever you know has fat in it, halve it. For instance, if you order French fries, only eat half of them. Then triple the amount of fruits, vegetables, and grains that you have with that food. Replace food that has fat with food you adore that doesn't."

so hungry that you start nibbling on it while you read the menu.

Try not to do this. If it's boring white bread, ask the waiter to take it away; you don't really want to waste your calories on something that tastes like cotton, do you? But even if the bread looks absolutely wonderful, try to hold off till you've read the menu. If you opt to order light—maybe an appetizer and salad—go ahead and enjoy the bread. But if you know you're going to order a big entrée and are apt to eat a good deal of it, hold off on the starchy stuff and save your appetite (and calories) for the main event. If you do reach for the rolls, don't reach for the butter—those calories are *definitely* better expended elsewhere.

Appetizers and Salads

• If you have a fatal attraction to fatty appetizers, don't even look at that part of the menu—unless you want to make a meal of appetizers, as more and more people do. If you do go for a fat-laden choice, stick with just one, plus a salad. Or share a couple with your dining companions.

• When possible, opt for steamed seafood or vegetable-based appetizers. Watch out for sauces, dips, and anything fried in batter.

• Order a cup rather than a bowl of soup, and choose those that are broth- or tomato-based. Or make a meal of a richer soup plus salad.

• Order your salad with dressing on the side, and dip your fork into the dressing before forking up some greens. You'll eat much less dressing this way, guaranteed. At salad bars, stick with the greens and raw veggies, with vinaigrette or low-fat dressing; otherwise your salad may end up with a fried dinner's worth of fat.

Entrées

• Order entrées with the fewest ingredients—grilled chicken instead of chicken pot pie, for example.

• Choose meat, fish, or poultry that is broiled, grilled, baked, steamed, or poached rather than fried. Broiled or grilled entrées are often basted with large amounts of fat, however. Ask to have your entrée prepared without added fat, or request that lemon juice, wine, or just a small amount of fat be used.

• Many restaurants serve meat in portions much larger than 3 ounces—as much as 6 to 10 ounces or more. If you have a choice, order a smaller portion. A "petite" filet mignon, for example, is about 4 ounces when cooked; a regular-size filet mignon is about 6 ounces cooked.

• Select lean cuts of meat—try to avoid the prime rib and spareribs. Trim away visible fat.

• Opt for pasta with primavera or tomato sauce.

• Order a vegetarian dish—but first make sure it's not loaded with fat.

Vegetables

Watch out for added butter and sauces. Choose vegetables seasoned with lemon, herbs, or spices rather than fat. Asian restaurants often offer great

F.Y.I.

Protein was named more than 150 years ago, from the Greek word *proteios,* meaning "of prime importance."

Menu Meanings

If menu items claim to be low-fat, "light," or "heart-healthy," you can believe it. The FDA now requires that restaurants' nutritional claims meet specific requirements, and customers must be given the appropriate nutritional information for these items when requested.

Here are some terms to watch out for if you're wary of fat and sodium overload:	Here are some good-guy terms that will prove helpful in restuarants and other situations:
Buttered or buttery	Grilled
Smoked	Baked
Fried, batter-fried, pan-fried	Broiled
Breaded	Stir-fried
Barbecued	Roasted
Creamy or creamed	Poached
In its own gravy, with gravy	Vegetable-based
Teriyaki	Light
Hollandaise	Braised
Creole style	Marinated
Au gratin	Oil-free
Scalloped or escalloped	Steamed

stir-fry combinations; their menus also frequently include a section of low-fat options, with vegetables that are steamed rather than sautéed in oil.

Dessert

First, ask yourself if you really *want* (as in really, really want) dessert. Do you have room left to fully

enjoy it? If the answer is yes, you know the rap:
The best choice is sorbet or a fruit-based dessert,
though not if it's glopped with heavy cream or a
rich sauce. Or just opt for a decaf or skim cappuccino. If you desperately want that chocolate
mousse torte, and you deliberately saved room for
it, go ahead—but split it with a friend. This is
where the term "have your cake and eat it, too"
comes from. You can enjoy every bite—just make
them dainty ones.

Beverages

If you order wine or cocktails, go easy. Order wine by
the glass instead of by the bottle. Tip: Dry table wines
have about half the calories of sweet table wines.

As an alternative, try a wine spritzer—half
wine, half seltzer—or mineral water with a twist.

Fast Food

There are worse things than fast-food meals. Contrary to popular belief, fast food does *not* equal
junk food. Most fast-food fare offers protein and
some vitamins and minerals. But that doesn't mean
it's a nutritional gold mine—far from it. It's generally lacking in calcium, vitamins A and C, and fiber,
and the exorbitant calorie, fat, and sodium content
more than outweighs the nutritional benefits.

But it's convenient, quick, and relatively
cheap—and it's almost impossible to avoid. Don't
worry; you don't need to. Just keep the following
guidelines in mind:

• Choose regular sandwiches rather than doubles
(or worse), and skip the extras: bacon, cheese,

STREET SMARTS

"As soon as you've
finished eating, put a
mint candy in your
mouth to signal the
end of the meal and to
help you resist further
temptation," advises
Brad Hughes, a twenty-
eight-year-old medical
researcher.

Big Bad Food

Fast food is going beyond big, into supercolossal territory. To attract customers, burger and pizza emporia are offering beefed-up portions, with beefed-up fat and calories to go with them. For example: Burger King's Big King gives you 75 percent more beef and 12 more grams of fat than a Big Mac. Hardee's Monster Burger offers two beef patties, three slices of cheese, and four strips of bacon for 970 calories and 67 grams of fat. Where your health is concerned, this does *not* constitute more bang for your buck.

and sauces. Feel free to load up on lettuce, tomatoes, and onions.

• Instead of burgers, try lower-fat grilled chicken or roast beef sandwiches.

• Steer clear of deep-fat-fried fish and chicken sandwiches or chicken "nuggets." They've got more fat and calories than a plain burger, and with cheese or tartar sauce, they're even worse news.

• Skip the fries, or if you must have them, order a small serving and split it with a friend. If there is no friend, order only fries and skip the sandwich—but count this as a fat-laden snack, not a meal.

• Choose iced tea (make sure it's not presweetened) or water instead of a soda or shake.

• Skip fast-food desserts; they're likely to be high in fat and sugar, and you can find better-tasting ways to spend your calories.

Eating on the Run

If you constantly find yourself fitting in meals or meal-replacing snacks while you're scurrying to and from work or meetings, running errands, or picking up the kids, you should first ask yourself: Is this really necessary? If you are able to adjust your schedule even slightly, you can probably find time for a sit-down meal instead of some of those grab-and-go gulps. And chances are you'll be better off for it, both nutritionally and mentally.

Impossible, you say? Then how about replacing some of those fast-food meals or convenience store and vending-machine goodies with healthy foods from home? Here are some suggestions:

• Small cans or cartons of fruit juice;

• Cut-up fresh fruits or vegetables;

• Whole-grain crackers and reduced-fat peanut butter or low-fat cheese;

• Raisins or dried fruit mix;

• Air-popped popcorn with onion or garlic powder;

• Low-fat pretzels.

No, they're not meals, but they'll tide you over until you can sit down and eat something substantial.

Snacking and Good-Time Eating

As you learned in chapter 6, there's nothing inherently wrong with snacking. In fact, done right, it can help keep your weight loss on track by stabilizing your blood sugar, and thus your energy level.

It's easy to come up with smart snack ideas that satisfy hunger and boost nutrition. That said, it's natural to crave high-fat, sugary foods when you first begin to cut down and replace them with healthier choices. And it's also natural to be tempted by the vast array of eating opportunities that await you at nearly every social, entertainment, or sports event.

Not to worry. By following the anti-deprivation guidelines in this book, you can enjoy any food you want, including the occasional high-fat or sugar-laden indulgence. This should go a long way toward eliminating those gnawing cravings for "forbidden" foods.

Still, it can be hard to maintain the moderation habit when you're constantly assaulted with snacking and nibbling opportunities. Ahead is advice on eating, drinking, and merrymaking without suffering a dietary hangover.

Fun Food

When you think about it, there are very few occasions or activities that *don't* involve food. Shopping, movies, ball games, celebrations, even work breaks—there's no escape. However, there are smart ways to deal with all the food temptations these events offer—and they don't all involve Just Saying No.

Just as with restaurant dining, if you plan ahead for a food-filled activity, and cut down before and after, you can eat pretty much anything you want—in moderation. This is a comforting thought, because not only is it difficult to say no to every delicious food that crosses your social path, but it's also very difficult to say no to a host who may get miffed if you don't eat up.

First, one overriding piece of advice: Always try to plan, at least to some extent, what you are going to eat—snacks included—over the course of a day. Factor in social events, movies, and other food-featuring activities. You plan other aspects of your day—why not this?

Here are some other tips to help in minimizing damage:

Parties and Business Functions

• Have a small snack or glass of juice before you leave for an event; you're more likely to overeat on an empty stomach.

• Bring your own fresh fruit or vegetable platter, along with a couple of low-fat dips. Hover nearby.

• Beware of hors d'oeuvres. They go down easy and add up fast. Limit yourself to the two best-looking ones.

• Keep a glass of seltzer in your hand so you have something to sip on; it'll help keep you from grabbing at random snacks just to keep your hands busy.

• At a buffet, give all the selections the once-over before you start filling your plate. Then choose only the best two or three.

• At a sit-down dinner, you'll probably have no control over what you're served, *and* you'll feel obligated to eat it. This is a tough one. If you tell your host you're a vegetarian (whether it's true or not), you're likely to end up with the healthier menu items. In any case, don't let yourself feel pressured to eat more than you want; if worse comes to worst, you can always feign illness!

SMART MONEY

Getting the right food mentality is difficult. Remember these words of wisdom from Michael Fumento, medical journalist and author of *The Fat of the Land.* "Food should not be your friend. Food is sustenance, and sometimes it's entertainment. But never, never make it your friend. People should be your friends, pets should be your friends, books should be your friends."

• If you're hosting a dinner party, wrap up the leftovers and give them to guests to take home. Or freeze individual portions to eat later.

• If it's your birthday, don't pass up your own birthday cake! Just choose a moderate piece.

Movies, Shopping, Vacations, Outings, and Other Distractions

• If you're going to the movies and determined to avoid the temptations of Raisinets or that deadly movie popcorn (a medium tub offers over 850 calories and 52 grams of fat), bring along your own healthy snacks so you won't feel deprived when everyone else is munching away. Or choose the best options at the concession stand: Buy a box of minimally harmful Junior Mints and grab a handful, then give the rest of the box to your companion; or go with Twizzlers, which are significantly lower in fat and calories than many other candy choices. If only popcorn will do, sneak in your own air-popped version. Or order a small bag of the "real thing," enjoy every bite, and cut back on your fat intake for the rest of the day.

• If you're grazing at a street fair or at the mall, use your nutritional know-how to choose foods that are fun but not fatally so—a bagel instead of fried dough, low-fat frozen yogurt instead of a sundae.

• Watch out for vacation syndrome—the certainty that overcomes you, whenever you venture away from home, that the rules of healthy eating no longer apply. You should feel free to ease up and enjoy yourself—no one expects you to measure portions on vacation—just don't go overboard to the extent that you'll come home laden not only with souvenirs but several new pounds—and a big load of guilt.

Choose your indulgences with care; they're more enjoyable that way. For example, if you're in New Orleans and can't live without a fried shrimp po'boy glopped with dressing, don't hesitate! But don't order a regular soda instead of your usual diet soda, merely because you're on vacation.

If you've been on a well-balanced, non-deprivation eating plan up until your trip, you'll find it much easier to avoid going overboard.

Snacking in Solitude

There's no place like home for an eating binge. That's because it's the place where there are fewest distractions—and thus there is the greatest chance for boredom and loneliness. It's also where you have the easiest access to food. It's just a few steps away—and it's easy enough to sneak it when no one's looking.

The best way to avoid excess snacking, then, is by keeping temptation at bay. That means filling your kitchen with only healthy treats and plenty of them—popcorn, low-fat crackers, sorbet, and the

The Truth about Late-Night Eating

Contrary to popular myth, food you eat at midnight will not fatten you any more than the same food eaten at noon. It does not matter, calorie-wise, *when* you eat. It's true that your metabolism slows down before you go to sleep, but your body will draw on that food for energy tomorrow, if not tonight. A big meal before bedtime may make it hard to get to sleep, but that's about it.

Late-night eating is a bad idea because it tends to be non-hunger-related. Chances are, if you continue eating after dinner, you're doing so because you're bored, tired, stressed out, or just craving something to chew on. Often that means a lot of calories you don't need.

Nibble Alert

In a study at the Obesity Research Center at St. Luke's–Roosevelt Hospital in New York, researchers found that ten obese subjects who were unable to lose weight on 1,200 calories a day were actually eating about 1,000 calories more daily than they had estimated because of their nibbling.

If you nibble while preparing meals, try sipping water or seltzer, chewing gum, or preparing a plate of carrot and celery sticks to keep close at hand. If you're tempted by leftovers, ask someone else to perform cleanup duties. Or brush your teeth before you tackle them—it reminds you that eating time is over.

like—that you can turn to when the munchies strike. If none of these does the trick, you'll at least have to go to the store to assuage your craving. Says Kelly Streit, M.S., R.D., a nutritionist in private practice in Portland, Oregon: "If you have to work at indulging, it buys you time to think about what you're doing. You may decide to make do with a healthier version of what you're craving—or realize you can go without a treat at all."

If you do go shopping for treats, think small. While it's true that nutritious snacks can't always satisfy your yen for candy, potato chips, or other salty, sugary, fatty treats, a small taste of what you crave may be enough. Many a candy urge has been satisfied by a bite-size chocolate bar. Whatever you do, don't bring home any low-nutrition treat in multiple-serving size. "Availability creates craving," says psychologist Stephen Gullo, president of the Institute for Health and Weight Sciences in New York City and author of the book *Thin Tastes Better.* Gullo recommends forgoing even a semi-innocent pint of sorbet in favor of individual servings: "You'll end up eating less."

Trigger Foods

If there are certain foods you know you can't eat without going out of control—so-called trigger foods—you have two choices: Try to avoid them altogether, or eat them only in controlled situations. The second option is preferable, since it will allow you to enjoy that food instead of living in fear of it.

By all means, if you worship at the altar of chocolate cake, do not bake one and tell yourself you'll only have one slice. Don't even give yourself that temptation. If you are craving cake, buy a single-serving piece at a restaurant or a bakery. If you miss baking, go ahead and bake a cake, and bring it to a friend (maybe she'll offer you a slice!).

When Healthy Eating's Not a Family Affair

If you're surrounded by family members who subsist on high-fat foods, you've either got to exert tremendous self-control or—preferably—start changing their habits. Work- and time-intensive as it is, try to do the grocery shopping and meal planning whenever possible. And try weaning them gradually from their usual heavy fare by making small substitutions: Use half as much meat in casseroles and stews; substitute ground turkey for ground beef; make vegetarian versions of favorite dishes. If you sometimes cook high-fat favorites for your family, take a small portion for yourself and fill the rest of your plate with vegetables and grains.

Educate your family about the risks associated with high-fat foods. Of course, this might not make much of an impact on your kids, so try telling them that eating well will improve their

It can be very easy to make rationalizations when you are trying to lose weight. Cassandra Lowry, a forty-three-year-old retail sales associate, has some good experience here: "I had the following *misconceptions:* If you eat something when no one sees you, the calories don't count; when you eat with someone else, the calories don't count if you don't eat more than they do; foods eaten for medicinal purposes—for example, hot choco-late,cheesecake—never count; cookie pieces contain no calories because breakage causes calories to leak out; food you order for your kids will have no calories if you finish it to keep it from going to waste."

sports performance, make their hair shinier—whatever hits home with them.

What to Watch For

Lots of parents have a habit of "cleaning the plate" when kids don't finish their food. It's all well and good to avoid waste, but not when it goes to your waistline: You can easily add another 300 or so calories to your daily total with your plate-cleaning ways.

Another syndrome to watch for: the tendency to eat as much as your mate (or date, for that matter). It's easy to fall into the habit of matching your dining companion bite for bite, but if your companion is male, it's a sure route to bulking up. The average American woman eats about a third less calories than the average American man, according to recent government surveys, so if you're a woman, aiming to consume about two-thirds as much as your man is probably wise.

If your family is rife with junk-food fanatics and your dietary hints fall on deaf ears, your best bet is to keep their food out of your sight. Put it in a separate cabinet or in the bottom corner of the refrigerator.

The Lowdown on Drinking

Everyone is aware of the dangers of alcohol: It's a strong psychoactive substance, it's very toxic, and it can easily lead to addiction.

What's easy to forget (even before you've had a

drink or two) is that alcohol is also a potent source of calories. A regular beer's about 150 calories; a glass of wine about 105; a mixed drink can range from about 155 for a martini to 260 and beyond for piña coladas and other sweet concoctions. (A drink equals twelve ounces of beer, five ounces of wine, or one and a half ounces of 80-proof liquor.)

That said, light to moderate drinking probably won't do any harm to your health or your waistline. The important thing is to know what "light to moderate" means:

Light: You have a drink occasionally, usually when socializing or celebrating.

Moderate: You have a glass of wine, a beer, or a mixed drink most days, but not every day. More than this, on more than an occasional basis, qualifies you as a heavy drinker and puts you at risk for problems that extend well beyond weight gain.

To control calories and intake:

• Order drinks mixed with water or seltzer, not sweetened with soft drinks.

• Order a glass of wine rather than a carafe.

• Try a wine spritzer (wine and seltzer water).

• Try the "light" version of your favorite beer.

F.Y.I.

Many studies suggest that moderate alcohol consumption (no more than one drink a day for women and no more than two drinks a day for men) helps prevent heart disease. But for women, risk of heart disease remains low until menopause—so for premenopausal women, drinking has no known protective value.

Mood and Food

How often do you turn to food in times of stress, anger, boredom, or even elation? Maybe you can't answer that. Many people—women especially—confuse such emotions with hunger and never learn to distinguish between the two.

It's time to learn. Keeping a food diary (as discussed in chapter 2) will help you recognize the relationship between your mood and your eating habits. Once you see those patterns, you can start working to break them.

If you are stressed out or unhappy about a relationship, work, family, or any of the myriad complications in this stress-filled world, you need to learn other ways to cope with or solve your problems. Food is not going to do the trick. If you're bored or lonely, call a friend, pick up a book, listen to music, or, best of all, take a brisk walk. These solutions may sound simplistic, but you'll be surprised to find how easily you can thwart a mood-related binge by taking just one small action. The hard part is making yourself do so.

Of course, taking a walk isn't going to solve any major life problems. If you are seriously stressed or depressed, please think about talking to a therapist or counselor. It's easy to think of food as your one reliable companion in life, but as comforting as food can be in the short run, you know that it's not going to solve anything. Try reaching out to people, not food.

If you know you are prone to emotional overeating, it's especially important to keep tempting foods out of your reach. That way, if you do overeat, you'll be bingeing on healthy foods and thus keep the damage to a minimum. Or you'll put important stop-and-think time between you and the treats at the nearest store. But in the long run, it's essential to try to break this habit altogether.

THE BOTTOM LINE

You can control the contents of your kitchen (if you live alone, anyway), but there's a whole world of food and food-related situations that you have to master in order to stay the healthy course. Yes, there are temptations everywhere you look, but if you plan ahead, use your high nutritional IQ, and think in terms of moderation, not deprivation, you can face any menu, movie concession stand, or mood with confidence.

Weight Loss That Lasts

You may think losing weight is the hard part; perhaps you'll say "It's clear sailing from here" once you've adopted a healthier lifestyle and notice the pounds start peeling off. But although you should feel optimistic and confident, you should also be aware of the challenges still ahead. One of these is the infamous weight-loss plateau. Another is learning to maintain your weight loss over the long haul—a much greater, and longer-term, challenge than losing the weight in the first place. The good news: By following this book's guidelines for sensible, gradual weight loss and focusing on changing your habits and mindset rather than opting for a quick-fix diet, you've set the stage for a lifetime of healthy eating. And the longer you continue, the less effort you'll need to make to maintain your good habits; you'll simply want to eat right and exercise because it makes you feel so good.

Still, let's face it: It's easy, and tempting, to let your resolve lapse a bit once you've achieved your health or weight-loss goals. This chapter offers some tips and positive reinforcement to keep you on track.

Hitting a Plateau

Everything's been going along just fine—you've been eating a diet rich in nutritious, low-fat foods, keeping a careful eye on portions, and exercising regularly, and you've been losing a healthy one or one and a half pounds a week. Then, suddenly, your weight loss comes to a standstill. What's up?

You've reached a "plateau," a phenomenon well

known to everyone who's ever tried to lose weight—especially those who have done so time and again. The plateau signifies that your body has adjusted to your lower caloric intake and has slowed down your metabolism to conserve energy—because your body can't tell the difference between starvation and voluntary weight loss. Plateaus can be very frustrating, but remember: They're only temporary. Dos and don'ts for coping:

• Don't panic. Remember, this is a normal stage of weight loss.

• Don't lower your caloric intake even further. Your body will respond by slowing your metabolism even more, which does nothing to help your weight-loss goals.

• Don't weigh yourself every day. Obsessing about the numbers on your scale is not a healthy way to lose weight in any case, and it can be particularly discouraging during a plateau. Once a week is plenty.

• Do continue with your current eating plan. If you've been losing weight steadily, the plateau won't last for long; soon you'll resume losing at your previous rate.

• Do increase your exercise level. It's a great way to boost your metabolism and get your body off that plateau.

Adjusting Your Expectations

If you find yourself stuck in a permanent plateau, it's time to reevaluate your strategy and your goals. First, review your daily eating habits and make sure you're not "cheating" yourself by eating more (weigh and measure foods to be certain) and exercising less than you think you do.

If you can honestly say you're sticking to your plan, and you're still unable to lose weight, you should think about whether your target weight is really a realistic one for you. You shouldn't have to starve yourself in order to reach it. If you are eating and exercising healthfully and at a level that's comfortable for you, it may be time to declare success right where you are.

Knowing When to Stop

Everyone's heard the saying "You can never be too rich or too thin." The first half of that statement is arguable; the second is patently false. You can indeed be too thin—to the point where you endanger your health and even your life. For many overzealous dieters, it can be hard to know when to stop.

If you have reached the weight range you aimed for at the start of your weight-loss plan, but think you could stand to lose a few more pounds, please consult a doctor first. You may be in danger of developing an eating disorder such as anorexia nervosa or bulimia.

People suffering from anorexia nervosa have a distorted body image; they're unable to perceive themselves as anything but fat, no matter how emaciated they become. Bulimics frequently binge, purge, or fast to control their weight. Although both of these conditions are linked to psychological problems such as anxiety and depression, they can also be triggered by dieting. Sticking to a well-balanced, sensible weight-loss plan goes a long way toward preventing such dieting extremes. But there is no question that losing weight and keeping it off can easily become an obsession. If you think you may be developing an eating disorder, you should seek help immediately. Psychotherapy, sometimes combined with medication, can provide very effective treatment.

Keeping It Off

Weight-loss maintenance can be more difficult than weight loss itself for several reasons:

1. There's no structure. When you're starting to get fit and lose weight, you can find structure and support everywhere—books, magazines, counselors, trainers: All are happy to give you advice and guidance. But when you reach the maintenance stage, it's easy to feel set adrift. What now? Who's going to guide you through the rest of your life?

2. The thrill is gone. You set yourself a goal and achieved it. Whether you measured your progress by your scale or by your waistband, or merely by how much healthier and more energized you feel, your new lifestyle reaped noticeable improvements. Week by week, you amassed evidence of your success, and those incremental rewards

SMART MONEY

Don't let the number on the scale be your only measurement for success. Arizona-based weight researchers Susan Olson, Ph.D., and Robert Colvin, Ph.D., offer the following advice for when the scale shows no loss in pounds: "Weight loss is not an end in itself; it is the means to an end. . . . It is the means to more important goals." So stick with your program and don't let the scale discourage you.

inspired you to keep going. But now you're where you want to be, and there's no momentum to keep you motivated, no new notches to reach on your belt.

3. You want a break. Once you reach your goal weight, you'll naturally want to celebrate—and ease up a bit on your eating plan. That's fine. But you may have a hard time getting back in line if you stray too far off the healthy path.

4. You expected too much. If you resolved to lose weight with the conviction that thinness is the key to happiness, you're bound to be discouraged when you reach your goal.

Never fear: While these are very real concerns, they're eminently surmountable. Simply being aware of these potential problems—instead of expecting to land on easy street—will go a long way toward helping you tackle and overcome them. Read on for specific ways to cope.

Mapping Out a Maintenance Plan

It's true: There's no specific structured plan to follow once you've lost weight. Maintaining your weight loss involves only two simple "rules":

1. Find the right balance of calories and exercise to maintain your current healthy weight.

2. Keep eating the same healthy, low-fat foods that enabled you to lose the weight in the first place.

When you reach your target weight, not only should you celebrate, but you should also start adding calories to your daily intake. Hardly an onerous task! But you do need to be careful about how many calories you add, and where those calories come from. Eating a candy bar after lunch is not the right approach.

To maintain your weight, start by adding 200 calories, or one or two servings from the food pyramid, to your daily intake. An extra serving of grains is a great way to go. If you're still losing, add a serving of fruit or vegetables. It may take a little while, but eventually you will hit upon the right amount to keep you in fighting trim. You can eat these extra servings whenever you like, at meals or as snacks.

Remember that if you've been exercising, you'll need to stick with it. Otherwise the increase in calories might cause weight gain.

Working without a Net

While you may have turned to myriad sources of inspiration and instruction to guide you through your weight loss, ultimately no one but you was responsible for reaching your goals. In essence, you did it on your own. So although it may seem a bit daunting to enter the maintenance phase—which, after all, is a very long (lifelong) phase—without all the structure and support you might have received while losing weight, you have already armed yourself with all the knowledge and habits you need.

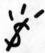

SMART MONEY

Weight-management expert at the University of Florida Michael G. Perri, Ph.D., offers this wisdom from his many years of experience: "Maintenance means much more than *weight* maintenance. It also includes the maintenance of other healthy lifestyle behaviors, such as healthy eating patterns, exercise, reducing stress, keeping healthy relationships, and more."

Staying Motivated

After you've reached your weight-loss goal—or any goal, for that matter—it's natural to feel triumphant. It's also natural, if less expected, to feel a little bit adrift. When you are in the process of losing weight, the rewards are tangible: Your clothes start fitting better, and soon you need new ones; you start feeling more energetic and healthy; people comment on how good you look. But once you've reached your target weight, those overt forms of positive reinforcement are no longer there.

What to do? Find new goals and new ways to keep yourself motivated, both fitness-wise and otherwise.

• If you find yourself gradually drifting away from your healthy ways, make an appointment with a nutritionist to bolster your food IQ and nip any bad habits in the bud.

• If your exercise routine is getting to be a yawn, make an appointment with a personal trainer at your gym; he or she can not only teach you new techniques but also bolster your workout resolve.

• Get together with other people—friends, neighbors, coworkers—who have recently lost weight and form a little moral-support group, reminding one another of how far you've come and bolstering one another's resolve to stay the course.

And take all that effort and attention you used to devote to your weight and start putting it into new activities and endeavors. Delight in the fact that you no longer have to waste time obsessing about extra pounds, fad diets, or binge-and-starve cycles.

Giving Yourself a Break

Once you reach your goal weight, it's natural to want to take a little break from your healthy routine. Maybe you want to go out to a fabulous restaurant, eat whatever you please, and forget all about food groups and fat grams. Fine—do it! Even while you're trying to lose weight, and certainly after you've reached your goal, there's nothing wrong with an occasional blowout. But it should be a controlled blowout. Yes, there is such a thing.

A controlled blowout involves planning. You go out to the restaurant, eat what you want, and come home feeling satisfied and not one bit guilty. You're secure in your resolve to go right back to your healthy eating and exercise plan tomorrow. An *uncontrolled* blowout usually doesn't start with a plan, and usually doesn't stop at the end of a single meal—or maybe even a single day. And it usually has a lot less to do with food than with your emotional state.

Bouncing Back from a Lapse

In some ways, it can be even more difficult to recover from a binge *after* you've achieved your goal weight than it was during the process. For one thing, you no longer have that forward momentum working for you. And for another, it's possible you may feel a little uncomfortable with the new, trimmed-down you. Although you're healthier, more energetic, and happier with your appearance than you were before, it's a big adjust-

SMART MONEY

"Once I dropped to a normal weight for my size, I had to come to terms with another common obsession: wanting to have a perfect body. I had to convince myself that I could be the best possible me without wanting to look like a fashion model. . . . Of course I could be thinner. I could stop snacking on cereals, bread, and pretzels. I could refrain from splurging from time to time on ice cream or frozen yogurt. But in doing so, I could also risk the return of my old fixations on unhealthy foods and of the unwanted pounds that used to drag me down mentally and physically."—Jane Brody, "Personal Health" columnist, *The New York Times*

ment, and now and then it may be tempting to slide back into the old familiar, overweight you.

Don't let it happen. If you find yourself sitting, spoon in hand, in front of an empty ice cream carton, here's the wrong thing to do next: Start tearing your hair out and then proceed to devour everything else in the vicinity. Instead:

• Remind yourself how much you've achieved and all of the work you put into reaching your goals. And remind yourself, too, that one little lapse does not spell dietary doom.

• Go brush your teeth. Then go out for a walk, call a friend, turn on some music, or meditate. Do something to get your mind off the lapse and back on a positive track.

• Don't feel guilty. Allowing yourself the occasional lapse is crucial. Maintain that all-important sense of balance and flexibility. If you eat something not-so-great today, balance it out by eating fewer fatty or sugary foods tomorrow. And be sure to get in a workout: It's one of the best ways to put yourself back in a positive, I'm-in-control frame of mind.

Reality Check

Of the many fallacies surrounding weight loss, the most harmful one is this: Losing weight will change your life. If you embark on a weight-loss and exercise plan in the firm belief that you will, upon achieving your goals, emerge as a whole new person, you are bound to be disappointed.

Losing weight is not going to win you undying love, get you the job of your dreams, or give you inner peace. Maybe it won't make you look like a beauty pageant winner, either. What it will do, besides improve your health and help you look and feel your best, is give you a sense of self-empowerment. Use it to tackle other problem areas in your life. Start to reach out to people instead of food. Get involved in new endeavors and activities that will further bolster your self-esteem.

Of course, it's great to look your best, but what's really important is having the optimal health and energy to enjoy life. Now you have it; so get out there and enjoy!

A Final Note

Never stop congratulating yourself for achieving your goals. Losing weight and getting fit is an enormous achievement, and you'll reap the rewards for the rest of your long, healthy life. Cheers!

THE BOTTOM LINE

Losing weight isn't the end of the story. After you've worked so hard to achieve a svelte and healthy physique, you've got to figure out how to maintain it. Yes, it still takes effort; sometimes it can be the hardest part of the battle. But because you've been smart enough to nix the get-thin-quick schemes in favor of a sane, sensible, livable eating plan, you've made things easy on yourself. Count yourself among the weight-loss champs who've learned to enjoy food without letting it control them.

Appendix: Calories and Fat for Selected Foods

Food	Amount	Calories	Fat (in grams)
Breads, Cereals, and Grains			
Breads and Crackers			
Bagel	3-inch	163	1
Bread, Italian	1 slice	85	0
Bread, pumpernickel	1 slice	82	1
Bread, whole wheat	1 slice	67	2
Cracker, graham, low-fat	2 whole	110	2
Cracker, saltine	5	60	2
Muffin, bran	1 small	112	5
Muffin, corn	1 small	125	4
Muffin, English	1 whole	133	1
Pancake	1 small	60	2
Roll, hard	1	155	2
Cereals			
Bran flakes	1 cup	135	1
Cheerios	1 cup	110	2
Chex	1 cup	111	0
Granola, low-fat	⅓ cup	110	2
Grape-Nuts	⅓ cup	136	0
Oatmeal, cooked	1 cup	150	3
Puffed rice, plain	1 cup	50	0
Raisin bran	1 cup	174	1
Shredded wheat	1 biscuit	80	0
Total	1 cup	100	1
Wheaties	1 cup	101	1

Food	Amount	Calories	Fat (in grams)

Grains

Food	Amount	Calories	Fat
Barley, cooked	1 cup	195	1
Bulgur, cooked	1 cup	150	0
Couscous, cooked	1 cup	200	0
Macaroni, cooked	1 cup	183	1
Noodles, cooked	1 cup	213	2
Popcorn (air-popped)	1 cup	25	0
Pretzel, thin	1	24	0
Rice, brown, cooked	1 cup	216	2
Rice, white, cooked	1 cup	264	1
Rice cake	1	35	0
Wheat germ	2 tbsp.	15	0

Fruits

Food	Amount	Calories	Fat
Apple, medium	1	81	1
Applesauce, unsweetened	½ cup	53	0
Apple juice	1 cup	116	0
Apricot, fresh	1	17	0
Apricot, dried	¼ cup	77	0
Banana, medium	1	105	1
Blueberries	1 cup	81	1
Cranberry juice	1 cup	144	0
Grapefruit	½	37	0
Kiwi	1	45	0
Melon, honeydew	1 cup	60	0
Nectarine	1	67	1
Orange, medium	1	62	1
Orange juice	1 cup	112	1
Papaya	1 cup	55	0
Peach	1	37	0
Pear, Bartlett	1	98	1

Food	Amount	Calories	Fat (in grams)
Pineapple	1 cup	76	1
Plum	1	36	0
Prunes, stewed	½ cup	106	0
Raisins	¼ cup	109	1
Raspberries	1 cup	60	1
Rhubarb	1 cup	26	0
Strawberries	1 cup	45	1
Tangerine	1	37	0
Watermelon	1 cup	51	1

Vegetables

Food	Amount	Calories	Fat (in grams)
Asparagus, cooked	½ cup	22	0
Beans, green, cooked	½ cup	22	0
Beets, cooked	½ cup	26	0
Broccoli, cooked	½ cup	23	0
Brussels sprouts, cooked	½ cup	30	0
Cabbage, raw	1 cup	16	0
Carrot, medium	1	31	0
Cauliflower, cooked	½ cup	15	0
Celery, raw	1 stalk	6	0
Eggplant, cooked	½ cup	23	0
Kale, cooked	½ cup	21	0
Lettuce	1 cup	10	0
Mushrooms, cooked	½ cup	21	0
Okra, cooked	½ cup	34	0
Onion, cooked	½ cup	30	0
Peas, green, cooked	½ cup	63	0
Pepper, green, cooked	½ cup	12	0
Potato, white (with skin)	1 medium	220	0
Potato, sweet (no skin)	1 medium	118	0
Radishes	10	7	0
Spinach, raw	1 cup	12	0
Spinach, cooked	½ cup	20	0

Food	Amount	Calories	Fat (in grams)
Squash, acorn, cooked	½ cup	42	0
Squash, zucchini, cooked	½ cup	15	0
Tomato	1	24	0

Dairy

Cheese

American	1 oz.	106	9
Blue	1 oz.	100	8
Brie	1 oz.	95	8
Cheddar	1 oz.	114	9
Cottage, low-fat	1 cup	164	2
Feta	1 oz.	75	6
Gouda	1 oz.	101	8
Monterey Jack	1 oz.	106	9
Muenster	1 oz.	104	9
Parmesan	1 oz.	129	9
Provolone	1 oz.	100	8
Ricotta, part skim	½ cup	170	10
Swiss	1 oz.	107	8

Milk

Skim	1 cup	90	1
1 percent	1 cup	102	3
2 percent	1 cup	121	5
Whole	1 cup	150	8
Buttermilk	1 cup	99	2

Yogurt

Plain, nonfat	1 cup	127	trace
Plain, low-fat	1 cup	144	4
Plain, whole	1 cup	139	7

Food	Amount	Calories	Fat (in grams)

Meat, Poultry, Eggs, Seafood, and Legumes

Meat (cooked)

Food	Amount	Calories	Fat (in grams)
Bacon	1 slice	36	3
Beef, ground (lean)	3 oz.	230	15
Beef, bottom round	3 oz.	178	7
Beef, sirloin	3 oz.	165	6
Beef, top round	3 oz.	153	4
Ham	3 oz.	140	6.5
Lamb, leg	3 oz.	162	7
Pork, center loin	3 oz.	204	11
Pork, tenderloin	3 oz.	141	4
Veal, rib	3 oz.	150	6
Veal, top round	3 oz.	128	3

Poultry (cooked)

Food	Amount	Calories	Fat (in grams)
Chicken, white meat	3 oz.	142	3
Chicken, drumstick	3 oz.	151	5
Chicken, thigh	3 oz.	163	7
Turkey, white meat	3 oz.	115	1
Turkey, dark meat	3 oz.	137	4

Eggs

Food	Amount	Calories	Fat (in grams)
Egg, large	1	75	5
Egg white, large	1	16	0
Egg yolk, large	1	59	5

Seafood (all cooked except canned items)

Food	Amount	Calories	Fat (in grams)
Catfish	3 oz.	129	7
Cod	3 oz.	89	1
Flounder	3 oz.	99	1

Food	Amount	Calories	Fat (in grams)
Halibut	3 oz.	119	3
Mackerel	3 oz.	171	9
Monkfish	3 oz.	82	2
Orange roughy	3 oz.	75	1
Salmon, Atlantic	3 oz.	175	11
Salmon, Coho	3 oz.	151	7
Salmon, pink, canned	3 oz.	114	5
Snapper	3 oz.	109	2
Surimi (imitation seafood)	3 oz.	84	1
Swordfish	3 oz.	132	4
Trout	3 oz.	128	5
Tuna, fresh	3 oz.	156	5
Tuna, canned in water	3 oz.	90	1

Shellfish

Food	Amount	Calories	Fat (in grams)
Clams, canned	3 oz.	126	2
Crab, king	3 oz.	82	1
Lobster	3 oz.	84	1
Oysters	3 oz.	116	4
Scallops	3 oz.	75	1
Shrimp	3 oz.	84	1

Legumes (all cooked except tofu)

Food	Amount	Calories	Fat (in grams)
Beans, black	½ cup	125	1
Beans, garbanzo	½ cup	143	1
Beans, lima	½ cup	94	0
Beans, navy	½ cup	129	1
Beans, pinto	½ cup	117	0
Lentils	½ cup	115	0
Split peas	½ cup	116	0
Tofu	3 oz.	88	6

Food	Amount	Calories	Fat (in grams)

Fats, Oils, and Salad Dressings; Nuts and Seeds

Fats and Oils

Food	Amount	Calories	Fat (in grams)
Butter	1 tbsp.	102	12
Cooking spray	1 spray	1–7	0–1
Margarine	1 tbsp.	102	11
Mayonnaise	1 tbsp.	99	11
Mayonnaise, low-calorie	1 tbsp.	40	4
Oil, corn	1 tbsp.	120	14
Oil, olive	1 tbsp.	120	14

Salad Dressings

Food	Amount	Calories	Fat (in grams)
Blue cheese	1 tbsp.	77	8
Blue cheese, low-calorie	1 tbsp.	10	1
French	1 tbsp.	67	6
French, low-calorie	1 tbsp.	22	1
Italian	1 tbsp.	69	7
Italian, low-calorie	1 tbsp.	16	2
Thousand Island	1 tbsp.	59	6
Thousand Island, low-calorie	1 tbsp.	24	2

Nuts and Seeds

Food	Amount	Calories	Fat (in grams)
Brazil	¼ cup	230	29
Cashew, dry roasted	¼ cup	197	16
Macadamia, oil roasted	¼ cup	240	26
Peanuts, oil roasted	¼ cup	210	18
Peanut butter	1 tbsp.	94	8
Pistachio, dry roasted	¼ cup	185	16
Pumpkin seeds, roasted	¼ cup	72	3
Sunflower seeds, oil roasted	¼ cup	208	20
Walnuts	¼ cup	190	18

Source: United States Department of Agriculture and individual food manufacturers

Note: Calories and fat grams vary by brand. Check nutrition labels.

Index

Adzuki beans, 106
Aerobic exercise, 18
Aerobics and Fitness
  Association of America, 21
Agriculture Department, U.S.
  (USDA), 86, 112
  Food Guide Pyramid of, 80-
  110, 135-36
Alcohol, 48, 147, 156-57
Alert eating, 10-11, 133
Almonds, 104, 105
Alternate diet/binge eaters, 39
Amaranth, 91
American Council on Exercise,
  21
American Dietetic Association,
  37
Amino acids, 56, 57-58
Anasazi beans, 106
Anorexia nervosa, 162-63
Antioxidants, 66, 88
Appetite, 4, 6-7, 75, 77
Appetizers, in restaurants, 144-
  45
"Apple" shape, 32
Attitude, 2-5, 7, 14-15
Avocados, 97

Banana smoothie, 132
Basal metabolic rate (BMR), 8,
  36
Beans (dried), 58, 61, 76, 82,
  84, 104, 106, 176
Beef, 101-2. See also Meat
Beer, 157
Beta-carotene, 66
Beverages, 136
  alcoholic, 48, 147, 156-57
  juices, 92, 93, 94, 133
  in restaurants, 147, 148
Bioelectrical impedance, 33-34
Biotin, 67
Black (turtle) beans, 106
Blood pressure, 74, 75
Body fat. See Fat (body)
Body mass index (BMI), 29-31,
  34
Bok choy, 94-95

Bone density, 72, 73-74
Bottled products, in pantry, 120
Bran, 76, 89
Brazil nuts, 104, 105
Bread baskets, in restaurants,
  143-44
Breads, 61, 76, 81, 84, 85,   86,
  87, 88-89, 135, 171
Breakfast, 128, 137
Broccoli and broccoli rabe, 95
Brown rice, 90
Brown sugar, 62
Buckwheat, 91
Buddy system, 15-16, 166
Buffets, 151
Bulimia, 162, 163
Burgers, fast-food, 148
Business functions, 151-52
Butter, 108

Caffeine, 73, 137
Calcium, 69, 70, 72-74, 97, 98
  best sources of, 100
Calories, 34-37
  burned in various activities
    (chart), 19
  daily need for (chart), 34-35
  defined, 48
  everyday cooking and, 125-27
  from fat, percent of, 51-52
  labels and, 114-15, 118, 119
  metabolic rate and, 8, 36
  minimum intake of, 135
  recommended reduction in,
    37
  in reduced-fat foods, 54-56
  in selected foods (charts),
    171-77
Cancer, 30, 49, 66, 76, 81,   88,
  92, 97
Canned goods, in pantry, 120-
  21
Cantaloupe, 93
Carbohydrates, 52, 59-62
  calories in, 48
  complex, 60-62, 88-90, 116,
    131
  diets high in, 60

fiber and, 75-76
high-protein diets and, 57, 59
labels and, 116
recommended intake of, 60
simple, 60-62
Cardiovascular disease, 25, 30,
  49, 50, 53, 66, 76, 88, 92,
  115, 157
Center for Nutrition Policy and
  Promotion (USDA), 86
Cereals, 61, 81, 84, 87, 89,   99,
  171
Change:
  incremental approach to, 85
  weight loss and, 168-69
Cheese, 81, 84, 99-100, 125, 174
Chicken, 84, 102, 124, 142, 175.
  See also Poultry
Chickpeas, 106
Chocolate, 109-10
Cholesterol (blood), 50, 51, 53,
  115
Cholesterol (dietary), 50, 53-54
  labels and, 115, 118
Citrus fruit, 92-93
"Cleaning the plate," 156
Cocktails, 147
Cocoa, hot, 132
Complex carbohydrates, 60-62,
  88-90, 116, 132
Consumer Response Center
  (FTC), 42
Cooking, 122-27
  flavor secrets for, 124
  reducing fat in, 125-27
  sources on, 123, 126
Cooking Light Magazine, 123
Copper, 70
Cottage cheese, 100
Cross-training, 22
Cruciferous vegetables, 97, 98

Dairy products, 53, 57, 81-82,
  84, 85, 86, 97-101, 125,   135,
  174
  adding to diet, 99
  best bets, 97-101
  see also Cheese; Milk; Yogurt

Denial or deprivation, 3, 136
  moderation vs., 11-13
Desserts, 60, 94, 134, 146-47, 148
Diabetes, 30, 88, 134
Diaries, of eating and exercise, 37-41, 158
Diet and Weight Loss Home Page, 3
Dieting, 3, 5-7, 25
  high-protein diets, 57, 59
  metabolic rate and, 6, 13, 14, 59
Dinner menus, 130
Dinner parties, 151-52

Eating:
  alert, 10-11, 133
  food diaries and, 37-41, 158
  mood and, 39, 157-58
  patterns of, 38-39
  in restaurants, 140-48
  on the run, 148-49
  slowly, 11, 137
  timing of, 10, 153
Eating disorders, 162-63
Eating Well, 123
Educating yourself, 5-7, 46-47, 62
Eggs, 53, 57, 82, 84, 102-3, 125, 175
Emotional eating, 41, 157-58
Energy, 48, 134.
  See also Calories
Entrées, in restaurants, 145
Essential fatty acids, 48, 51
Evaporated skim milk, 99, 125
Exercise, 16-22
  bone density and, 73-74
  and calorie-burning in various activities (chart), 19
  cholesterol level and, 53
  enjoyment factor and, 19-20
  everyday activities and, 21
  intensity of, 18
  in maintenance, 164, 166
  plateaus and, 161
  set point and, 17
  sources on, 21
  variety in, 22
  weight training, 20-21
Expectations, 162, 164, 168-69

"Extra lean," on labels, 118

Fad diets, 5-7
Fast food, 147-48
  alternatives to, 148-49
Fat (body), 29, 32-33, 49, 57, 59, 60, 134
  body mass index and, 29-31
  distribution of, 32, 34
  measuring, 33-34
Fat-counter guides, 52
"Fat-free," on labels, 118
Fat-free foods, 50, 53, 54-56
Fats (dietary), 48-56, 82, 107-9, 135
  calories and fat grams in (chart), 177
  cholesterol and, 53-54
  down side of, 49
  everyday cooking and, 124-27
  fat-free or reduced-fat foods and, 50, 53, 54-56
  good vs. bad, 49-51
  labels and, 114-16, 118
  need for, 48-49
  recommended intake of, 50, 51-52, 107-8
  reducing intake of, 108-9
  in selected foods (charts), 171-77
  very-low-fat diets and, 52
Fat substitutes, 55
Federal Trade Commission (FTC), 42, 43
Fiber, 61, 75-76, 88
  foods rich in, 98
  labels and, 116, 119
Figs, 94
Fish and seafood, 53, 57, 82, 84, 103, 175-76
  in restaurants, 142, 145
  shopping for, 120
Flavor, 124, 141
Folic acid, 67, 93
Food diaries, 37-41, 158
Food Guide Pyramid, 80-110, 134-35
  number of servings and, 83-86
  serving sizes and, 82, 84, 103, 114
  smart foods in, 87-110
"Fresh," on labels, 119

Fries, fast-food, 148
Frozen foods, 121
Fruits, 53, 61, 76, 81, 83, 84, 85, 86, 90-94, 135, 172-73
  adding to diet, 94
  A (C, etc.) list, 98
  best bets, 92-94
  dried, 94
  phytochemicals in, 69
  shopping for, 117, 120
Frying, alternatives to, 123-24
Fun food, 150-53

Garbanzo beans, 106
Genetics, 7
Glucose, 59, 60
Glycogen, 60
Goal-setting, 8-9, 10, 162
  in maintenance, 166
"Good source of," on labels, 119
Grains, 58, 61, 87, 88-90, 172
  exotic, 91
Grazing, 10, 133-35

Habit, eating out of, 9-10
HDLs (high-density lipoproteins), 52
"Healthy," on labels, 119
Healthy eating, 11, 112-58
  cooking and, 122-27
  daily do's and don'ts for, 137
  desserts and, 134
  dieting vs., 3
  drinking and, 156-57
  focusing on, 4-5
  fun food and, 150-53
  guidelines for, 135-36
  menus for, 127-31
  mood and, 157-58
  other family members and, 155-56
  restaurant meals and, 140-48
  shopping and, 112-22
  small meals and, 133-35
  snacks and, 129, 132-33, 149-50, 153-54
  trigger foods and, 154-55
Heart disease. *See* Cardiovascular disease
Herbs, 121
"High," on labels, 118, 119

Honey, 62
Hors d'oeuvres, 151
Hunger, 4, 6-7, 133, 153
 emotional eating vs., 157-58
 listening to your body and, 9-11
Hydrogenated fat, 50
Hydrostatic weighing, 33
Hypertension, 74
Hypoglycemia, 134

Ice cream, 100-101
Indulgences, 109, 153, 167
International Food Information
 Council, 86
Iodine, 70
Iron, 71, 101, 104
"Irradiated," on labels, 119
Isometrics, 21

Juices, 136
 fruit, 92, 94
 vegetable, 93, 133

Kale, 95
Kamut, 91
Ketosis, 59

Labels, 112-19
 claims on, 116, 117, 118-19
 "Nutrition Facts," 112-17
Lapses, 167-68
Lasagna, 123
Late-night eating, 153
"Lean," on labels, 118
Lentils, 106
"Light" or "lite," on labels, 119
Linoleic acid, 51
Linolenic acid, 51
Listening to your body, 9-11
"Low," on labels, 118
Lunch menus, 129

Maintenance, 163-69
 lapses in, 167-68
 "rules" for, 164-65
 staying motivated in, 166-67
Malls, eating in, 152
Manganese, 71
Margarine, 108
Marinades, 125
Meat, 47, 53, 82, 84, 85, 86, 101-
 2, 104, 135, 175

cooking, 125-27
 in restaurants, 142, 145
 shopping for, 120
 trimming visible fat from, 125
Meat loaf, low-fat, 123
Menus, 127-31
 breakfast, 129
 checklist for, 136
 devising your own, 135
 dinner, 131
 lunch, 130
 sample, 128-31
Metabolic rate, 25, 36
 defined, 8
 dieting and, 6, 13, 14, 59
 plateaus and, 161
Mexican red beans, 106
Milk, 57, 73, 81, 84, 85, 86, 97-
 98, 99, 100, 124, 136, 174. See
 also Dairy products
Millet, 91
Minerals, 64, 69-74
 labels and, 116-17
 supplements and, 68-70
Mineral water, 73, 100
Moderate eaters, 38
Monounsaturated fat, 50-51,
 108, 115
Mood, 9, 26, 49
 emotional eating and, 39, 157-
 58
Motivation, 4, 6, 27
 in maintenance, 166-67
Movies, eating at, 152
Mung beans, 106
Muscle, 13, 29
 weight training and, 20-21

Niacin, 66
Nibbling, while preparing
 meals, 154
"Nonfat," on labels, 118
Nutrition, 46-110
 carbohydrates and, 59-62
 cholesterol and, 53-54
 educating yourself about, 5-6,
 46-47, 62
 fats and, 48-56
 fiber and, 75-76, 88
 Food Guide Pyramid and, 80-
 110, 135-36
 minerals and, 64, 69-74

protein and, 56-59
 sources on, 47, 86, 108
 vitamins and, 64-69
 water and, 75, 77-78
Nutritional claims:
 on food packages, 116, 117,
 118-19
 on restaurant menus, 146
"Nutrition Facts" labels, 114-
 17
 calories from fat per serving
 in, 114-15
 carbohydrates, fiber, and sugars in, 116
 fat, cholesterol, and sodium
 in, 114-15
 % Daily Value in, 115, 116
 protein in, 116
 serving size, servings per container, and calories per serving in, 114
 vitamins and minerals in, 116-
 17
Nuts, 82, 84, 104-5, 177

Oatmeal, 76, 89
Oils, 50, 82, 107, 108, 125, 177
Olestra, 55
Overweight:
 criteria for, 30
 genetics and, 7

Packaged goods, in pantry, 120-
 21
Pantothenic acid, 67
Pantry, well-stocked, 120-21
Parties, 151-52
Pasta, 61, 81, 82, 84, 87, 145
Patience, 3, 13
Peanut butter, 105
"Pear" shape, 32
Pecans, 104, 105
Percent body fat test, 33-34
% Daily Value, 115, 116
Phosphorus, 71
Physical activity, 21
 diary of, 37-41
 see also Exercise
Phytochemicals, 69
Plateaus, weight-loss, 160-63
Polyunsaturated fat, 50-51, 108,
 115

Portions. *See* Serving sizes
Potassium, 71, 75
Potatoes, 58, 61, 83, 124
Poultry, 53, 57, 82, 84, 102, 104, 125, 142, 175
  removing skin from, 126
  in restaurants, 145
  shopping for, 122
Protein, 56-59, 73, 97, 101-7
  best bets, 101-7
  calories in, 48
  complete vs. incomplete, 57-58
  diets high in, 57, 59
  enhancing intake of, 107
  labels and, 116
  recommended intake of, 56, 57
  vegetarian diet and, 58-59
  worst bets, 105
Pumpkin seeds, 104, 105

Quinoa, 91

Rebound weight gain, 13, 14, 25
Recommended Daily Allowances (RDAs), 57, 69, 73
"Reduced," on labels, 118, 119
Reduced-fat foods, 50, 54-56
Restaurant meals, 140-48
  appetizers and salads in, 144-45
  beverages in, 147
  bread baskets in, 143-44
  desserts in, 146-47
  entrées in, 145
  fast-food, 147-48
  menu meanings and, 146
  strategies for, 142-43
  vegetables in, 145-46
Restrained eaters, 38
Riboflavin, 65
Rice, 61, 81, 84, 90
Root vegetables, 61, 117

Salad bars, 120-21, 144-45
Salad dressings, 108, 177
  in restaurants, 142, 144
Salads, 96, 144-45
Salmon, Pacific, 103
Salt. *See* Sodium

Sandwiches, fast-food, 147-48
Saturated fat, 49, 50, 51, 108, 115, 116
  cholesterol level and, 53-54
  labels and, 118
  recommended limit on intake of, 51, 52
Sauces, 127, 142
Scale watching, 8-9, 29, 161, 163
Seafood. *See* Fish and seafood
Seeds, 104-5, 177
Selenium, 72
Servings:
  number of, 83-86
  per container, 114
Serving sizes:
  in Food Guide Pyramid, 82, 84, 103, 114
  labels and, 114
  in restaurants, 142, 145
Sesame seeds, 104, 105
Set point, 17
Shopping, 15, 112-22
  for fresh food, 117-22
  pantry items and, 120
Simple carbohydrates, 60-62
Skin-fold calipers, 33
Skipping meals, 137
Small meals, 132-34
Snacks, 129, 149-50, 151
  healthy, 131-32
  low-fat or nonfat, 90
  in solitude, 153-54
Social occasions, 150-53. *See also* Restaurant meals
Sodas, 136
Sodium (salt), 72, 73, 74-75, 142
  labels and, 115, 118
Soups, 144
Sources, 3, 9, 21, 37, 42, 47, 52, 58, 86, 108, 123, 126
Soy milk, 98
Spelt, 91
Spices, 121
Starches, 87. *See also specific starches*
Starvation mode, 6, 13
Stevia, 61
Strawberries, 93
Street fairs, 152
Strength training, 20-21
Stress, 26, 157-58

Substitutions, 12
Sugars, 60, 62, 107, 109
  labels and, 116, 119
  replacing fat with, 55
Sugar substitutes, 61
Supplements, 68-69
Support system, 15-16, 166
Sweet potatoes, 95
Sweets, 82
Swimming, 22

Target weight, 8-9, 10, 162
Thiamin, 65
Thirst, 77
Thyroid, 14
Tofu, 104-6
Tomatoes, 96
Trans fats, 50, 51
Trigger foods, 154-55
Triglycerides, 52
Tums, 100

Unrestricted meal overeaters, 39
Unsaturated fat, 49, 50-51, 108, 115

Vacations, 152-53
Vegetable juices, 93, 132
Vegetable proteins, 57-58, 103-7
Vegetables, 53, 61, 73, 76, 81, 83, 84, 85, 86, 90-92, 135, 173-74
  adding to diet, 96
  A (C, etc.) list, 98
  best bets, 94-97
  cruciferous, 97, 98
  phytochemicals in, 69
  in restaurants, 142, 145-46
  shopping for, 117, 120
Vegetarianism, 58-59, 145
"Very low," on labels, 118
Vitamin A, 48, 65, 66, 69, 98
Vitamin B_1 (Thiamin), 65
Vitamin B_2 (Riboflavin), 65
Vitamin B_3 (Niacin), 66
Vitamin B_6, 66
Vitamin B_{12}, 66
Vitamin C, 66, 67, 98
Vitamin D, 48, 68, 69
Vitamin E, 48, 66, 68, 69, 88
Vitamin K, 49, 68

Vitamins, 64-69
  labels and, 116-17
  supplements and, 68-69

Waist-to-hip ratio, 32, 34
Walking, 22
Water, 59, 75, 77-78, 76
  retention of, 8, 74
Weighing yourself, 8-9, 29, 161, 163
Weight:
  evaluating, 27-34
  healthy ranges for, 27-28
  set point and, 17
Weight loss:
  attitude and, 2-5, 7, 14-15
  bad times for, 25-26
  calorie intake and, 34-37, 62, 133
  eating disorders and, 162-63

educating yourself and, 5-7, 46-47, 62
exercise and, 16-22
factors to consider before, 24-27
fat intake and, 51
focusing on what you *should* eat in, 78
food and exercise diaries in, 37-41, 158
going it alone vs. with group, 42-44
life changes and, 164, 168-69
listening to your body and, 9-11
maintaining, 160, 163-69
moderation vs. denial in, 11-13
motivation for, 4, 6, 27
pace of, 13-14
plateaus in, 160-63

portion control and, 82, 103
right reason for, 26-27
setting goal for, 8-9, 10, 162
support system and, 15-16
water intake and, 77
Weight-loss centers, 43-44
Weight training, 20-21, 29
Wheat germ, 89, 90
White beans, 106
Wild rice, 90
Willpower, 4, 7
Wine, 147, 157
Work, exercising at, 21

Yogurt, 73, 81, 84, 174, 98-99, 100, 125
Yo-yo dieting syndrome, 6, 9, 25

Zinc, 72, 101
Zone, The, 57

Books in the
Smart Guide™ Series

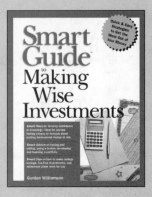

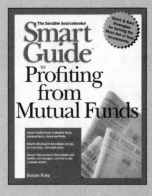

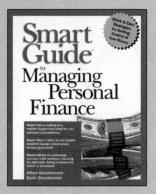

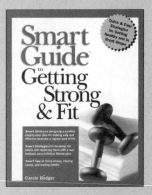

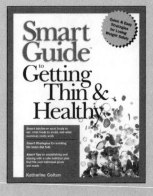

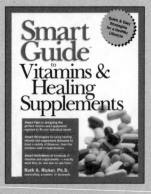

Smart Guide™ to
Getting Strong and Fit

Smart Guide™ to
Getting Thin and
Healthy

Smart Guide™ to
Making Wise
Investments

Smart Guide™ to
Managing Personal
Finance

Smart Guide™ to
Profiting from Mutual
Funds

Smart Guide™ to
Vitamins and Healing
Supplements

Available soon:

Smart Guide™ to
Boosting Your Energy

Smart Guide™ to
Healing Foods

Smart Guide™ to
Home Buying

Smart Guide™ to
Relieving Stress

Smart Guide™ to
Starting and Operating
a Small Business

Smart Guide™ to
Time Management